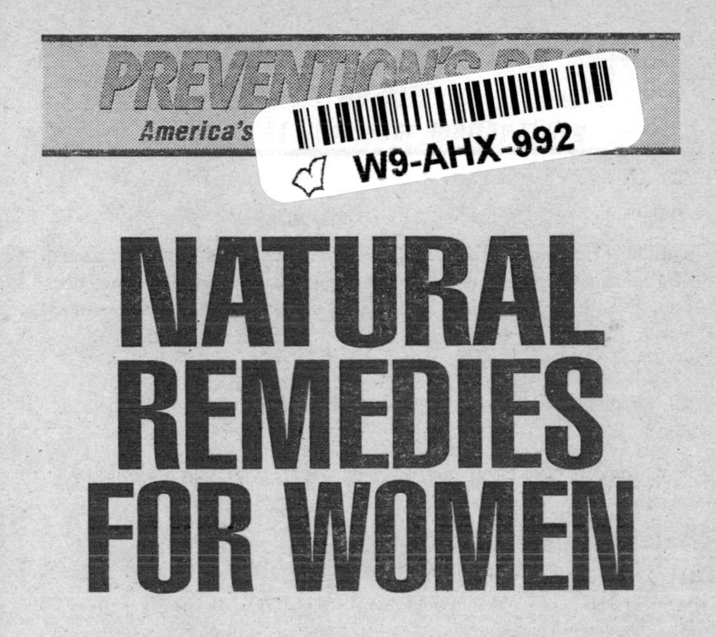

NATURAL REMEDIES FOR WOMEN

By the Editors of *Prevention* Health Books

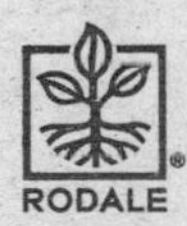

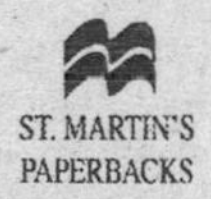

ST. MARTIN'S
PAPERBACKS

If you purchased this book without a cover, you should be aware that this book is stolen property. It was reported as "unsold and destroyed" to the publisher, and neither the author nor the publisher has received any payment for this "stripped book."

Notice

This book is intended as a reference volume only, not as a medical manual. The information given here is designed to help you make informed decisions about your health. It is not intended as a substitute for any treatment that may have been prescribed by your doctor. If you suspect that you have a medical problem, we urge you to seek competent medical help.

The information in this book is excerpted from *Natural Remedies* (Rodale Inc., 1999).

Prevention's Best is a trademark and *Prevention* Health Books is a registered trademark of Rodale Inc.

NATURAL REMEDIES FOR WOMEN

Book Designer: Keith Biery
Cover Designer: Anne Twomey

0–312–97503–1 paperback

Printed in the United States of America

Rodale/St. Martin's Paperbacks edition published July 2000

St. Martin's Paperbacks are published by St. Martin's Press, 175 Fifth Avenue, New York, NY 10010.

10 9 8 7 6 5 4 3 2 1

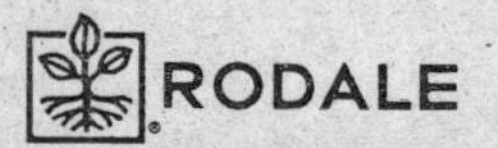

WE INSPIRE AND ENABLE PEOPLE TO IMPROVE
THEIR LIVES AND THE WORLD AROUND THEM

Board of Advisors

JoAnn E. Manson, M.D., Dr.P.H.
Associate professor of medicine at Harvard Medical School and codirector of women's health at Brigham and Women's Hospital in Boston

Mary Lake Polan, M.D., Ph.D.
Professor and chairperson of the department of gynecology and obstetrics at Stanford University School of Medicine

Elizabeth Lee Vliet, M.D.
Founder and medical director of HER Place: Health Enhancement and Renewal for Women and clinical associate professor in the department of family and community medicine at the University of Arizona College of Medicine in Tucson

Lila Amdurska Wallis, M.D., M.A.C.P.
Clinical professor of medicine at Weill Medical College of Cornell University in New York City, past president of the American Medical Women's Association (AMWA), founding president of the National Council on Women's Health, director of continuing medical education programs for physicians, and master and laureate of the American College of Physicians

Carla Wolper, R.D.
Nutritionist and clinical coordinator at the Obesity Research Center at St. Luke's/Roosevelt Hospital Center in New York City and nutritionist at the Center for Women's Health at Columbia Presbyterian Eastside in New York City

Contents

Part Three: Your Body

Part Four: Your Mind

Introduction

Want to be on the forefront of the twenty-first century health revolution?

Then bone up on the natural remedies in this book—and start taking charge of your own health.

The 1990s saw American women embrace natural healing in astounding numbers. Since 1990, use of herbal remedies in the United States has increased 380 percent, and use of vitamins for healing has risen 130 percent—figures, by the way, that come from that bastion of traditionalism and mainstream medical practice, the *Journal of the American Medical Association*. That magazine's beliefs were once the antithesis of natural healing.

But things are changing.

Today the majority of U.S. medical schools offer courses in alternative medicine. And more and more highly regarded medical centers, such as the University of Pennsylvania Medical Center in Philadelphia and Beth Israel Medical Center in New York City, are opening integrated medicine centers where treatments combine alternative and traditional approaches.

All that is good news, but there's another trend that is even more interesting: People prefer to treat themselves. That's why they find natural remedies so appealing.

The natural therapies that people are more often using include herbs, vitamins, folk remedies, homeopathy, massage, and self-help groups. People most frequently use them to treat chronic conditions, such as back problems, headaches, depression, and anxiety.

The information you'll find in this book was culled from interviews with more than 100 of the nation's leading practitioners of natural healing. Every piece of advice was double-checked to ensure its accuracy and your safety.

Even natural medicine can have side effects, so please read the precautions in the Safe Use Guidelines on page 263 before treating yourself. And if you're pregnant or under medical care for any problem, it's a good idea to check with your doctor before taking any natural supplements.

PART ONE

Feel Your Best

Soothe Everyday Annoyances

Headaches. Backaches. Hives. A lot of us can't seem to get through a day, let alone a week, without some minor health nuisance interfering with our lives. But consider yourself lucky. There are dozens of easy ways to solve life's little health glitches.

"Many health problems respond very well to self-care," says Jill Stansbury, N.D., assistant professor of botanical medicine at the National College of Naturopathic Medicine in Portland, Oregon, and a naturopathic physician in Battle Ground, Washington. And many of the most successful self-care techniques are home remedies that have existed for decades, passed down through generations of caregivers.

Got a cold? Sure, the modern home remedy—cough syrup—works just fine. But you might find out that the century-old technique of drinking marshmallow tea works even better.

And there's no doubt that over-the-counter antihistamines can do wonders for the itching of hives. But if you want to bypass drugs altogether, try what your great-great-grandmother probably did—an oatmeal bath.

To find the best remedies, we interviewed caregivers and doctors for successful solutions to the most vexing minor health problems. Here are the top picks for solving everyday annoyances.

Aches and Pains

Most sudden (what doctors call acute) pain involves muscles—particularly muscles that are weak, tense, or in spasm. They crowd and irritate neighboring nerves, which registers as discomfort or dull pain somewhere in your body.

It may sound contradictory, but you can often avoid pain simply by making those muscles work harder. Research into sports medicine has shown that stretching and movement help keep muscles flexible. And they benefit not only the muscles but the joints that they serve as well. Muscles that are flexible increase the range of motion of the nearby joints. This improves the flow of synovial fluid, the joint's lubricant, which nourishes the joint and reduces or prevents pain.

But even the best-oiled machine needs some tinkering from time to time. So when you get that ache-all-over feeling, here's what to do.

Add ginger to your bath. Sprinkle 2 tablespoons of powdered ginger into a tub of warm water, then climb in for a 20-minute soak. The ginger-water combination creates a sensation of heat, which helps relieve pain.

Gently stretch away soreness. Yoga, with its gentle stretching movements, can help ease and even prevent most body aches. Practice the following sequence.

- Stand with your arms over your head and your feet shoulder-width apart. Bend to the left, exhaling as you do. Hold for 3 seconds, then inhale as you return

The 10 Best Hiccup Cures

1. Place a spoonful of granulated sugar under your tongue and let it dissolve.
2. Gently rub the back of your throat with a soft swab.
3. Pull on your tongue.
4. Put a little ice on the skin around the front of your throat, just above your collarbone.
5. Chew papaya digestive tablets (available at health food stores) or a slice of fresh papaya or pineapple.
6. Make yourself sneeze by sniffing a dash of pepper.
7. Slowly sip a glass of ice water.
8. Hold your breath for 30 seconds.
9. Breathe into and out of a paper bag.
10. Pull your knees into your chest and lean forward.

to an upright position. Do the same to the right side. Repeat three or four times, alternately bending left and right.

- Still standing with your feet shoulder-width apart, place your hands on your lower back and lift your chest. Gently bend backward, inhaling as you do. Hold for a few seconds, then return to an upright position. Exhale on your way back up. Repeat three times.
- Stand with your hands on your lower back and your feet shoulder-width apart. Bend your knees slightly and lean forward as far as is comfortable, exhaling as you do. Hold for 3 seconds, then return to an upright position, inhaling as you straighten up. Repeat three times.

Chill it out. For muscle strain that is painful but not debilitating, apply ice wrapped in a towel to the affected area. Leave the ice in place for 20 minutes for large muscles (such as those in the back), 10 to 15 minutes for small muscles (such as those in the elbows and calves), and 5 minutes for painful muscles in the face, hands, or feet. Repeat six times a day—three of those times in the evening—until the pain is reduced by half.

Bad Breath

Bad breath is another universal complaint. Fiery and odorous foods, such as garlic, are obvious causes. Not so obvious: *not* eating. If you avoid mouthwatering meals, you may naturally decrease the amount of saliva, which fights odor-causing bacteria in your mouth. Some women find that their breath seems more malodorous around the time of their periods. Bad breath can also be the sign of impending gum disease.

Popping a breath mint or swishing mouthwash masks the problem but doesn't eliminate it. The following remedies freshen your breath naturally.

Have an after-dinner drink of water. Simply swishing a mouthful of water around your mouth after eating can deter bad breath. As a bonus, it helps wash away plaque, the sticky buildup of bacteria and tartar that leads to tooth decay and gum disease.

Go for the garnish. That sprig of parsley you find on the diner's blue plate special has a history and a purpose. A few nibbles are enough to vanquish stale breath. Parsley is a rich source of chlorophyll, which is a powerful breath freshener. If you don't like the taste, try parsley capsules instead. They're available in drugstores and some supermarkets.

Sip a cup of tea. Brew four whole cloves and 2 tablespoons of crumbled-up cinnamon sticks in 1 quart of water. Bring to a boil, cover, and simmer for 5 minutes. Remove the pot from the heat and let the tea steep for 20 minutes. Strain, allow to cool, and drink. Both cloves and cinnamon are potent antiseptics that can dissipate bad breath.

Blisters

As painful as a blister can be, it serves a very important purpose. It acts as a natural bandage, protecting the wound underneath from infection. And the fluid inside keeps the skin moist, so the wound heals quickly.

Blisters on the hands usually result from the friction generated during activities like raking and sweeping. In most cases, they're best left intact, but sometimes they're so large and uncomfortable that popping them is the only way to provide relief. Or they may open on their own.

With that in mind, here are the basics of blister care that you can use wherever blisters appear.

Pop properly. If you decide to pop a blister, first sterilize a needle with the flame of a match or with rubbing alcohol. Then prick the "bubble" at the lowest point on your body. That way, gravity helps to drain the fluid and relieve pressure.

Save your skin. Whether you pop a blister or it breaks open on its own, leave that little flap of skin in place. It provides protection for the wound underneath.

Keep it clean. Gently wash the blister with soap and water. Use liquid soap if it's available; bar soap may be coated with bacteria from previous uses.

Wrap it up. Once you have cleaned the blister, cover it with a bandage. This not only keeps out dirt and germs but also provides a comfortable cushion against friction. If your blister is open, coat it with a first-aid antibiotic ointment such as Mycitracin or Polysporin before applying the bandage. (Pure aloe vera gel can also help heal blisters because it contains both anti-inflammatory and antibiotic properties. It is sold in drugstores.)

Bloating

For women, one of two things is to blame for bloating—water or air. During your menstrual cycle, your body's supply of the hormone progesterone drops off in the 7 to 10 days before your period. Your body responds by storing salt, which in turn leads to water retention.

But bloating can also result from air that is either swallowed when you eat or produced in your digestive tract by high-fiber foods.

Here's what you can do.

Step out for a stroll. Walking or other light exercise dispels gas and alleviates that feeling of distension.

Drink dandelion tea. For premenstrual bloating, dandelion tea helps the body eliminate excess water. To make the tea, add 1 teaspoon of dandelion (either the root or the whole herb) to a cup of boiling water. Let steep for 5 minutes, then strain and allow to cool. Drink a cup of the tea two or three times a day.

Note: Women who are taking diuretics—for high blood pressure, for example—should not drink dandelion tea. And if you have gallbladder disease, you should not use dandelion without your doctor's okay.

Just add water. Consuming more liquids can actually reduce premenstrual bloating by diluting sodium in the body. Aim for a minimum of eight 8-ounce glasses of water a day.

Choose foods carefully. Certain foods produce a lot of gas and, therefore, contribute to bloating. Be wary of raw vegetables, cabbage, and beans.

Body Odor

Sweat has no odor, but it provides a moist breeding ground for bacteria. These bacteria eventually mix with a milky secretion from the apocrine glands, which are concentrated in the hairy areas under the arms and around the genitals. It's this brew that's responsible for body odor.

Most people can control body odor with a daily shower and deodorant. For those times when you need a little extra artillery, these strategies can help.

Lather up. Remember, body odor occurs only when bacteria mix with the secretion from the apocrine glands.

Wearing Last Night's Dinner?

When we eat certain foods and spices, our bodies extract some of the proteins and oils that give the food its particular scent, says Lenise Banse, M.D., director of the Northeast Family Dermatology Center in Clinton Township, Michigan. As part of the normal digestive process, these smell-producing compounds remain in the body's excretions and secretions for hours—and sometimes days—afterward. Fish, cumin, curry, and garlic are the biggest offenders.

Most of these same foods also leave strong cooking smells in the air that can cling to your hair, skin, and clothing and then linger on. So be sure to air out your kitchen if you don't want these smells to follow your guests out the door, advises Dr. Banse.

If your body starts to take on the odor of a food you haven't eaten, it could be cause for concern, says Dr. Banse. Fishy-smelling urine, for example, can be a sign of kidney trouble, and breath that smells like alcohol could indicate diabetes. See your doctor.

So you can minimize odor by using an antibacterial soap to cleanse the areas where the apocrine glands are concentrated—namely, under the arms and around the genitals. Once a day should do it.

Buy the right deodorant. For your underarms, choose an antiperspirant/deodorant combination that has aluminum chlorhydrate as its active ingredient. Such products minimize moisture, so bacteria have no place to grow.

Add cornstarch. Applying cornstarch to odor-prone areas also minimizes moisture and discourages bacterial growth. (Avoid using baby powder or talcum powder because use of these products in the genital area has been linked to ovarian cancer.)

Canker Sores

These craterlike sores—yellow at the base and red at the edges—can show up almost anywhere inside your mouth. No one knows for certain what causes them or why some people get them and others don't. For many women, stress and the menstrual cycle seem to be factors.

Left untreated, a canker sore usually goes away on its own in about 2 weeks. In the meantime, it can make routine activities such as talking and eating difficult and painful. To speed up the healing process, heed this advice.

Try a little Tea-L-C. Tannin, a compound in tea, seems to reduce the pain associated with canker sores. Soak a regular tea bag in warm water for a few minutes. Then squeeze out the excess water and place the tea bag directly on the canker sore for about 5 minutes. Repeat two or three times a day.

Watch what you eat. Certain fruits and vegetables—especially citrus fruits—are highly acidic, which can make a canker sore hurt more. Spicy foods can also aggravate pain. And some nuts, especially walnuts, can trigger an allergic response that leads to a canker sore.

Consider unexpected sources. Many people get canker sores as an allergic response to chewing gum, mouthwashes, menthol cigarettes, lozenges, and common medications such as aspirin and ibuprofen. If you seem to get a canker sore every time you put a certain something in your mouth, you're better off avoiding it.

Dry Mouth

Older people who are taking medications often experience dry mouth. But the condition can affect any person at any age, for any number of reasons.

For instance, you can get dry mouth simply by breathing through your mouth rather than your nose—such as when you're congested or under stress. More seriously, dry mouth can be a symptom of Sjögren's syndrome, an autoimmune disease that strikes women much more frequently than men. In addition, people who have diabetes are at increased risk for dry mouth, as are people who have undergone radiation therapy for head and neck cancer.

Combating dry mouth requires a two-pronged approach. First, you want to stimulate your salivary glands to put out as much "juice" as possible. Second, you want to compensate for any saliva shortfall. Here's what you need to do.

Get your jaw going. Chewing sugarless gum jump-starts saliva production while moistening the inside of your mouth. If you're not a gum fan, any chewy food will do.

Pick up a lemon drop. Sucking on a sugarless lemon drop activates the salivary glands. Or squeeze lemon into a glass of water, then drink up.

Stay wet with water. Carry a water bottle with you and sip every 10 minutes or so. The water helps keep your mouth moist and fresh. Steer clear of soft drinks and fruit juices. Without saliva to neutralize it, the sugar in these drinks can really do a number on your teeth.

Fever

A fever is not a disease. Rather, it's your body's way of protecting itself against invasive organisms, such as viruses and bacteria.

When you pick up a flu virus, for example, your immune system alerts your brain that it needs more heat in order to combat the virus. In response, your body temperature rises.

Truth be told, doctors don't agree on whether a fever requires treatment. The best advice: If it goes over 104°F, see your doctor right away. If it's under 104°F and making you miserable, by all means take steps to make yourself comfortable until your fever breaks. Here's what to do.

Make a splash. If you're hot and perspiring, draw a lukewarm bath and step in for a soak. Make sure the water is lukewarm, not cold. You don't want to get the chills.

Stay hydrated. As you perspire, you lose a lot of water. So be sure to keep your fluid intake up. Water is best, but fruit juices also help.

Get some rest. Your body demands rest while you have a fever. So stay in bed until your fever has been broken for at least 24 hours. Ask family and friends to pitch in with the cooking and laundry.

Flatulence

If flatulence weren't so downright embarrassing, we might be able to appreciate just how common it is. The average woman passes gas 12 times a day, the same as the average man.

Gender doesn't influence flatulence much, but eating habits certainly do. Ironically, many of the foods that are the most nutritious also produce the most gas: beans, broccoli, brussels sprouts, cabbage, cauliflower, corn, eggplant, garlic, onions, and radishes.

If the pressure builds, passing gas can be painful. But usually the discomfort is more social than physical. To put a stop to the sputtering, try these fast-acting tips.

Check out charcoal. Activated charcoal absorbs whatever is in your intestines, including gas and food particles that might later be turned into gas. Look for it in drugstores, and follow the label instructions for dosage.

Chew fennel seeds. Fennel helps to dissipate gas by relaxing muscle spasms in the digestive tract. Chewing ½ teaspoon of seeds is usually enough to leave you flatulence-free.

Pull the plug on pressure. To alleviate gas pressure in your lower abdomen, try this simple exercise. Lie on your back with your knees bent. Then alternately raise each knee toward your chest until you feel relief.

Break out the Beano. Beans have a reputation as the most potent gas producers around. You can render them gasless with a sprinkle of Beano. This liquid enzyme breaks down the indigestible sugars in beans. You can buy Beano in drugstores.

Hives

Hives are small, red, intensely itchy bumps that appear alone or in clusters on the surface of the skin. They occur when something causes cells to release an inflammatory substance called histamine.

That "something" could be just about anything, from

food to medication to stress. Even intense exercise or a hot shower can produce the dreaded tiny welts in people prone to them.

Hives usually go away on their own within a few hours. (If they don't, see a doctor.) In the meantime, these self-care measures can help stop the itch.

Apply ice. Rubbing an ice cube over the affected area for several minutes can actually help shrink the hives. Keep the cube moving so it doesn't freeze the surface of your skin.

Note: This remedy is not appropriate for anyone who develops hives when exposed to cold.

Sit in some oatmeal. Colloidal oatmeal effectively relieves the itching associated with hives. Following the package instructions, add the powder to a tub of lukewarm water, then climb in and soak for 10 to 15 minutes. Make sure that the water is lukewarm. Hot water can aggravate hives.

Stay cool, hang loose. Because heat can make hives worse, try to keep yourself as cool as possible. You'll also feel more comfortable if you wear loose-fitting clothes.

Pop a quercetin pill. If you get hives when you eat certain foods, try taking 250 milligrams of quercetin 20 minutes before eating them. A plant compound, quercetin has antihistamine properties, which may discourage outbreaks. Quercetin supplements are sold in health food stores and some drugstores, often in combination with vitamin C.

Muscle Cramps

A muscle cramp is your body's way of telling you that you have an imbalance of electrolytes. These substances keep cells functioning efficiently. The imbalance occurs when you don't have enough fluid in your system.

You can get a muscle cramp after exercising or overex-

Cramp, Cramp, Go Away

The quickest way to get rid of a cramp is to gently stretch out the muscle. For a cramp in the leg, try these stretches, suggests Rosemary Agostini, M.D., clinical associate professor of orthopedics at the University of Washington and staff physician at the Virginia Mason Sports Medicine Center, both in Seattle.

For a cramp in your calf, stand an arm's length (2 to 3 feet) away from a wall. Bend the knee of the non-cramped leg and step back with the other leg about 2 feet. Be sure to keep your back leg straight and both feet flat on the floor. Place your hands on the wall and bring your hips toward the wall while keeping your neck in line with your spine. Hold for 30 seconds, then stand up. After stretching out, massage or ice the affected area.

For a cramp in your hamstring (at the back of your thigh), sit on the floor with your cramped leg straight out in front of you. Bend your noncramped leg so that your foot is next to the knee of your cramped leg. Lean forward from your waist until you feel a stretch in the back of the thigh of the cramped leg. Hold for 20 to 30 seconds, then relax.

erting yourself and from not drinking enough fluid. When that happens, the muscles tighten and shorten.

A muscle cramp can also strike when muscles are fatigued from overwork. These cramps often occur hours after an activity—while you're sitting or lying down, for example.

With a little coaxing, a muscle cramp will usually uncramp itself in no time. Follow this advice.

Let your fingers do the working. When you get a cramp, your first instinct may be to rub the affected area.

And that's exactly what you should do. Gently massage the muscle until it relaxes.

Make nice with ice. Ice relieves pain and reduces inflammation. Try rubbing an ice cube over the affected area for 2 to 3 minutes. Or wrap an ice pack in a towel and lay it on the sore muscle for 20 minutes.

Turn up the heat. For some people, heat works better than ice in relieving a muscle cramp. Apply a heating pad for 20 minutes. If you don't have one, take a warm bath or shower instead.

Drink up. If you routinely get muscle cramps when you're active, chances are that you're not keeping yourself adequately hydrated. Remember to consume fluids before, during, and after any activity.

Sore Throat

We usually interpret a sore throat as a sure sign of an impending cold. Yet as often as not, something else is to blame. Dry air, dust, tobacco smoke, and misdirected stomach acid can dry out the mucous membrane that lines the respiratory airways. Even a marathon session of talking or cheering can leave throat tissues painfully raw and irritated.

With time and a little TLC, a sore throat usually gets better on its own. If your throat is extremely painful and you're having difficulty swallowing, see your doctor. You may have strep throat, which requires medical attention. To help ease the pain otherwise, try the following strategies.

Grab the saltshaker. Gargling with warm saltwater gently cleanses a sore throat and helps draw fluid from inflamed tissues. To make a saltwater rinse, mix ½ teaspoon of salt with 1 cup of warm water. Spit out the saltwater when you're finished. Repeat four or five times a day.

FOLK REMEDY: DOES IT WORK?

Honey for a Sore Throat

There's a good reason why Grandma would stir honey into a cup of steaming tea whenever her throat was feeling scratchy—honey kills bacteria.

"Honey is active against a wide range of bacterial and fungal species, many of which cause infections," says Angela Stengler, N.D., a naturopathic physician in Oceanside, California. "However, honey's antimicrobial effects would be so diluted after you swallow it that the honey probably couldn't kill bacteria throughout your whole body."

Yet honey is strong enough to kill some bacteria in your throat or at least soothe inflamed tissue there. Try stirring a teaspoon of it into a cup of hot tea or hot lemonade.

This remedy is safe for everyone except babies under 1 year of age. Honey contains dormant spores that are harmless to children and adults but may cause botulism in infants.

Recommendation: Worth a Try

Mend with marshmallow. No, not the sticky, sweet stuff. Marshmallow is an herb that quiets coughs and moistens and soothes a sore throat. To make a tea, place ¼ cup of dried, chopped herb (sold in health food stores) in a glass or a ceramic jar. Pour 1 pint of room-temperature water over the herb, then close the jar. Let the herb steep overnight. The next morning, strain the tea and add 4 teaspoons of honey. Sip ¼ to ½ cup of tea at a time over the course of the day.

Note: Marshmallow may slow the absorption of other medications taken at the same time.

Consider zinc. At the first sign of a sore throat, begin sucking on zinc gluconate lozenges. The tablets work best if you place them on your tongue and allow them to dissolve. These lozenges bathe throat tissues in a soothing zinc solution. You can buy zinc gluconate lozenges at health food stores and drugstores.

Avoid post-supper snoozing. Lying down too soon after a meal allows stomach acid to back up into your throat. The acid burns delicate throat tissues. This is one reason why you should eat your dinner no less than 4 hours before bedtime.

Tension Headache

Headaches are usually a by-product of stress. But stress is not the only cause. In fact, everything from blocked sinuses to skipped meals can trigger a tensionlike headache. In women, hormonal changes associated with menstruation or menopause are sometimes responsible.

A tension headache usually begins in the muscles at the back of your neck and slowly creeps toward your forehead. It may cause a throbbing sensation in your temples or behind your eyes.

Untreated, a tension headache usually subsides within a few hours. While an over-the-counter pain reliever can speed up the process, you may find that some of these natural remedies work just as well.

Draw the pain out with water. At the first sign of a tension headache, head for the nearest sink. Adjust the water temperature so that it's comfortably hot, then run your hands and wrists under the water for about 10 minutes. The heat draws blood away from your head and down into your hands, which may help relieve the pain.

Sniff a soothing scent. Keep on hand a bottle of peppermint essential oil (available at health food stores and bath-and-beauty shops). Then take a whiff straight from the bottle whenever a tension headache has you in its grip. The smell of peppermint short-circuits headache pain fast by improving circulation and drawing energy away from the pain.

Target your temples. Position your thumbs on either side of your head, right in the center of each temple. Using a firm, circular motion, massage your temples for a minute or two.

Schedule some tub time. Steep 2 tablespoons of lavender and 2 tablespoons of lemon balm in 1 cup of hot water for 10 minutes. Pour the tea into a tub filled with lukewarm water, then settle in for a 20-minute soak. You can buy both herbs in health food stores.

Fight Fatigue

Tired. Pooped. Drained. Weary. Exhausted. Those are just some of the adjectives people use to describe how they feel during a good part of their days. Some say they're tired when they get up in the morning. Others run out of steam in the middle of the afternoon. Still others feel so exhausted all day, every day, that they feel totally out of control of their lives.

For many people, the cause is obvious: They have too much to do and too little time to do it. "So many things demand our attention and pull us in different directions that our brains and bodies can't keep pace," says Susan Schenkel, Ph.D., a clinical psychologist in Cambridge, Massachusetts, and author of *Giving Away Success: Why Women Get Stuck and What to Do about It.*

Dr. Schenkel blames this kind of fatigue on what she calls stimulus overload. Unfortunately, a lot of people don't even recognize that they're overburdened. "They just accept what they're doing as normal," she explains.

Of course, plenty of other things can wipe you out. A poor night's sleep or a heavy meal can leave you dragging temporarily. More persistent, profound fatigue can be linked to stress, poor nutrition, lack of exercise, or even certain medications. It can also signal illness, such as iron deficiency anemia or problems with the thyroid gland.

Left to its own devices, fatigue can rob you of your lust for life. Don't let that happen. You can fight it and win.

If none of the following methods help and you've felt overwhelming fatigue for more than a month for no obvious reason, see your doctor. She can determine whether you have an underlying health problem that calls for medical treatment.

All-Purpose Energy Boosters

The amount of energy you have or don't have has a great deal to do with how you nourish your body and brain. The following habits, practiced daily, should keep you going and going all day long.

Get an extra 20 minutes of sleep a day. Either go to bed earlier, sleep later, or take a nap in the afternoon. Studies show that on any given day, half the men and women in the country are walking around sleep-deprived. On average, women need between 8 and 8½ hours of sleep a night, men 7 hours or so.

Delegate at least one chore to someone else. "Compared with men, women tend to place a lot more pressure on themselves," says Dr. Schenkel. "And if we finally do realize that we have to give up something, we feel guilty about it." So pick a chore and give it to someone else. Your body and brain will thank you.

Move your butt—and your arms and legs. It's a vicious cycle: The more exhausted you feel, the less you feel like getting out and walking the dog, gardening, or taking a stroll. But in an ironic twist of nature, the more you exercise, the less tired you'll feel and the more energy you'll have at the end of the day. So set aside 30 minutes a day, at least 3 days a week, for some kind of exercise, even if it's just walking.

Skip candy, cookies, baked goods, and other treats. Treats crowd out the nutritious foods your body needs, so you may be low on vital nutrients. The fat and sugar they supply wreak havoc with your metabolism and can leave you fatigued. And the extra calories pack on pounds, leaving you feeling like you're walking through mud, carrying a 25-pound sack of kitty litter.

Take a multi every day. Most of us don't always eat as well as we should. So take a multivitamin/mineral tablet that supplies 400 milligrams of magnesium and 25 milligrams of each B vitamin (including folic acid), nutrients needed to maintain energy.

Caution: People with heart or kidney problems should check with their doctors before taking supplemental magnesium. Supplemental magnesium may cause diarrhea in some people.

Your body needs magnesium to get energy from food. And deficiencies of B vitamins, especially B_{12}, have been linked to fatigue and memory loss, among other symptoms. Taking supplements with food will help you absorb them better.

Choose ginseng. Ginseng has long had a reputation as an energy enhancer, and new research seems to bear this out. The herb is sold in many different forms and potencies. Find a supplement that contains 100 to 125 milligrams of ginseng extract, standardized to contain 4 to 7 percent ginsenosides (the active ingredient in ginseng).

Note: Don't take ginseng without your doctor's okay if you have high blood pressure.

Become fluent in fluids. Water constitutes about 60 percent of your body weight. Dehydration can sap your energy and impair mental and physical performance. To ensure that you're well-hydrated, fill an empty 2-liter bottle with water every morning and take frequent sips throughout the day.

Afternoon Slump

You don't even have to look at the clock: You know precisely when it's 3:00 P.M. Your eyelids get droopy, your head starts to nod, and your entire body is begging to lie down for just a few minutes.

The urge to snooze in the mid-afternoon is altogether natural. As sleep researchers explain it, the human body is programmed for one long sleep period and one short sleep period every 24 hours. The short period occurs 12 hours after the halfway point of the longer period. So if you go to bed at 11:00 P.M. and wake up at 7:00 A.M., you'll likely feel sleepy around 3:00 in the afternoon.

To counteract a midday energy slump, women doctors recommend these quick pick-me-ups.

Stretch your legs. Nothing recharges your batteries better than exercise. So when you feel sluggishness setting in, lace up your sneakers and head out for a brisk walk around the block. Just 20 minutes of walking can energize you for up to 8 hours afterward.

Roll those shoulders. Shoulder rolls relieve tension and provide a quick energy boost. To begin, inhale, and squeeze your shoulders forward, as though you were collapsing your chest. Next, shrug your shoulders toward your ears. Then exhale and push your shoulders backward, moving your shoulder blades toward each other. Finally, drop your shoulders and relax.

Take a few deep breaths. Shallow breathing delivers less air to your lungs per breath, triggering changes that deliver less oxygen to your brain, heart, and the rest of your body. The result is grogginess.

To boost your energy stores, breathe in through your nose as deeply as you can. Hold for a few seconds, then breathe out, releasing the air slowly and deliberately.

Sample an energizing aroma. Put a drop or two of peppermint or rosemary essential oil on a handkerchief. Then sniff the scent for an on-the-spot lift. You can buy essential oils in health food stores and bath-and-beauty shops.

Focus on your feet. Use your knuckles to press on the center of the arch of one foot for a few seconds. Repeat on your other foot. According to practitioners of reflexology (the practice of stimulating different parts of the body via selected pressure points, usually on the hands and feet), stimulating this area of the foot wakes you up.

Capitalize on break time. For your afternoon coffee break, pair your cup of java with a high-carbohydrate food, such as three gingersnaps or four small fig bars. Caffeine provides a mental boost, while carbohydrates trigger the production of serotonin, a brain chemical that keeps you relaxed and focused.

Concentration Problems

Poor concentration could mean that you're bored with what you're doing. But it could also mean that you're too tired to pay attention. Here's how you can keep your thoughts on track.

Breathe in, breathe out. Besides boosting oxygen levels, deep breathing also dispels feelings of anxiety that can disrupt your concentration.

Get in tune with Bach. For some people, listening to baroque music seems to boost concentration. Research has shown that the works of German composer Johann Sebastian Bach are especially conducive to learning.

Eat often. Consuming frequent small meals keeps your blood sugar levels steady. And that keeps you clearheaded and sharp.

Select a smart snack. When your concentration begins to flag, eat a snack that pairs protein with carbohydrates—tuna on whole wheat bread, for example. The protein/carb combination helps sustain alertness.

Take a break. Sometimes poor concentration is your brain's way of telling you that you need a change of pace or a change of scenery or both. A quick walk around the block may be enough to shake off the cobwebs.

Think ginkgo. Research has shown that ginkgo biloba extract (GBE) improves concentration in people with cognitive deficiency, a condition caused by inadequate blood flow to and nerve damage in the brain. Look for a GBE product that's labeled "24/6." This tells you that the product contains 24 percent flavone glycosides and 6 percent terpenes. Take 120 to 240 milligrams of GBE in two or three separate doses every day. Keep in mind that the herb works slowly. Give it at least 8 weeks to do its stuff.

Insomnia

Do you have trouble falling asleep at night? Do you fall asleep just fine but wake up during the night and then find yourself unable to get back to sleep? Are you wide-awake hours before you need to be?

Roughly one-third of women have insomnia. Women seem to be especially prone to it, primarily because of hormonal changes that occur during menstruation, pregnancy, and menopause.

Here's how to relax your mind and body for sweet slumber when you want it.

FOLK REMEDY: DOES IT WORK?

Counting Sheep to Fall Asleep

It's the classic sleep-inducing vision: little white sheep, one by one, jumping over a fence.

Counting anything can help clear your mind of nagging thoughts and send you off to dreamland, says Susan Zafarlotfi, Ph.D., clinical director of the Institute of Sleep/Wake Disorders at Hackensack University Medical Center in New Jersey.

Counting and visualizing something pleasant—be it sheep, butterflies, or anything else—is a form of guided imagery, a practice that's known to help release stress and anxiety, notes Dr. Zafarlotfi. Counting sheep may be especially useful for women who often have trouble falling asleep because they're preoccupied with everyday worries and pressures.

Recommendation: Worth a Try

Get tea'd off. A number of herbs have properties that calm the nerves and foster sound sleep. Among the herbs to try are kava kava, St. John's wort, and valerian. To make a tea, add 1 tablespoon of dried herb to a cup of freshly boiled water. Allow the tea to steep for an hour, then strain and reheat before drinking. Drink a cup in the morning, one at noon, and one at night so that you're relaxed by the time you go to bed. Don't take valerian during the day, however, because it has a sedative effect. You can buy any of these herbs in health food stores.

Snooze in the afternoon. If your erratic sleeping pattern has really thrown you off schedule and you feel like you must nap, limit yourself to a half-hour snooze in the middle of the afternoon. If you sleep for more than a half-hour, your body will likely go into a deep-sleep phase that will leave you feeling groggy when you awaken.

Draw a bath. Soaking in a comfortably hot bath early in the evening causes your body temperature to rise. When you go to bed, your temperature quickly drops. This helps you fall asleep more easily.

Skip late-night noshing. Avoid eating a big meal less than 4 hours before bedtime. Otherwise, digestion—or indigestion—will keep you awake.

Exercise early. Working out may tire you out, but not in a way that's conducive to sleeping. Your body needs adequate time to recuperate from the exertion. Schedule your workout for at least 3 hours before bedtime.

Relax before retiring. Before going to bed, allow yourself at least 45 minutes of quiet time. Do some light reading (no suspense novels allowed), listen to soft music, or talk to your cat.

Create the right environment. Many people sleep best in a room that's on the cool side. So turn down the thermostat a few degrees before crawling between the sheets. Also, keep your bedroom dark and quiet.

Iron Deficiency Anemia

Iron deficiency anemia is most common among women, particularly those of reproductive age. The primary cause is menstruation. Menstruation depletes the body's supply of iron. When you run low on iron, your body produces fewer and smaller red blood cells. There is less hemoglobin, which means there is less oxygen floating around your bloodstream. This lack of oxygen leaves you feeling exhausted.

Mothers-to-be are prime candidates for anemia, as blood is diverted to the developing fetus and then lost during childbirth.

Some women become iron deficient not because of menstruation but because of poor eating habits. They're not consuming enough lean meats, legumes, and other iron-rich foods. Women who crash-diet are especially at risk.

While fatigue is a common symptom of iron deficiency anemia, it's not the only one. You may also experience shortness of breath, dizziness, lightheadedness, and poor resistance to infection. If you're tired and don't know why, see your doctor for proper diagnosis.

Anemia doesn't go away overnight. With treatment, you may feel better in a few weeks, but you'll need months to adequately replenish your iron stores. Visit your doctor again if you don't feel better after a month of treatment.

The following measures, in addition to any treatment your doctor recommends, can help you overcome anemia.

Feature meat at one meal. Meat is the richest source of iron and the primary source of heme iron, which is easily absorbed compared with the nonheme form found in plant-derived foods. Choose lean cuts such as flank steak, sirloin, and top round. Or buy cheaper cuts, such as strip steak and chuck steak, and trim the fat. Aim to eat one 3-ounce serving of beef a day.

Get juiced. Studies have found that vitamin C helps boost the absorption of nonheme iron found in plant-based foods. So when you're eating these types of foods, chase them with a glass of orange juice whenever possible.

Stock your iron stores. Most experts advise that you check with your doctor before taking iron supplements, to make sure that you actually need them. (Too much iron isn't always healthy either.) If you do need iron, take 300 milligrams of ferrous sulfate every day for 7 days only during menstruation. These supplements deliver the iron you need when you need it most, but without the risk of toxic buildup. They're available in drugstores without a prescription. Avoid taking them with milk or with food of any kind, which can actually inhibit iron absorption.

Shed the coating. If your doctor recommends iron supplements, look for a brand that is not enteric-coated. Your body can better absorb the iron from uncoated tablets.

Jet Lag

Flying across time zones may be exciting for the psyche, but it's exhausting on the body. That's because as your body greets a new day in a new place and new time, its internal clock remains set on the old time.

Generally, to reset its clock, your body requires 1 full day for every time zone crossed. In the meantime, you may experience an array of jet lag symptoms—not just sleep disturbances and fatigue but also headaches, digestive upset, and irritability. Interestingly, traveling from west to east seems to cause more problems than traveling from east to west because you're pushing your body's clock forward instead of back. Here's what to do to make jet lag a minor blip in your travel schedule.

Step outside. If you arrive at your destination during daylight, head outdoors for some light activity as soon as you can to give your body a chance to acquaint itself with the new time zone. The activity will help your body's natural time-keeping cycle adjust to your new schedule. A walk around the block is sufficient.

Spend time in the sun. Because the day/night cycle governs your body's clock, getting some sun exposure can expedite the adjustment. But you have to time it right. A good rule of thumb: If you fly from west to east, head outside in the morning and retreat indoors by late afternoon. If you fly from east to west, stay indoors in the morning and go outside in the late afternoon.

Follow the locals' lead. The first day in your destination, eat and sleep according to the new time, even if it's much earlier or later than your home time.

Be gentle to your digestion. Give your digestive system a chance to adjust to the new time zone too. At least at first, stick with light meals consisting of familiar foods. After a day or two, your stomach will be prepared should you decide to sample some more exotic fare.

Enjoy a java jolt. Caffeine can ease your body through the time zone transition, as long as you use it prudently. If you're flying from the West Coast to the East Coast, for example, have a cup of coffee with breakfast on the first morning in your destination. The caffeine can help compensate for the fact that you've essentially lost 6 hours of sleep. But don't rely on cup after cup of coffee to power you through the day, or you may find yourself the victim of caffeine overload.

Catch a catnap. If your body craves a nap, take one. Just make sure that your snooze lasts no longer than a half-hour.

Skip the cocktails. Alcohol affects your central nervous system and can interfere with sleep patterns. Wait a day to enjoy your bon voyage toast.

Conquer Colds and Infections

Germs. They're everywhere—on the phone, on the doorknob, and on the toilet handle. They travel home from the day care center, sail by you from a sneeze in aisle 11 at the supermarket, and shake your hand in the receiving line. They're in the air anyplace, anytime.

You can't avoid germs, but you certainly can resist them. The truth is that it's the strength of your immune system that determines whether you will or will not come down with the season's colds and flu.

Women are particularly prone to infections because they're inclined to put the needs of others above their own, explains Susanna Cunningham-Rundles, Ph.D., associate professor of immunology at the New York Hospital–Cornell Medical Center in New York City.

"There seems to be an attitude that if you're responsible for others, you're somehow stronger than everyone else and you don't have to worry about your health," says Dr. Cunningham-Rundles.

The first place to start building your immunity is right in the kitchen. "There's no substitute for eating right, and that means plenty of nutrition-packed foods like fruits and vegetables," says Dr. Cunningham-Rundles. She advocates incorporating something healthful into your diet before taking out something unhealthful. That way, changing your eating habits won't feel like punishment.

Supplement your diet with antioxidants—vitamins C and E and beta-carotene—which build up your immune system. This is especially important around the time of your period, when your immune system is more vulnerable to infection. Exercise builds immunity, so get out there and move for at least 30 minutes three or four times a week. And if you smoke, quit. Smokers are much more likely to get the flu or a respiratory infection than non-smokers. Finally, practice what you tell your kids to do: Wash your hands frequently throughout the day.

If the bug does get you, be sure to drink plenty of liquids, avoid rich foods (they're hard to digest), and get plenty of rest. Plus, you can speed recovery of specific infections with these natural remedies.

Bronchitis

Green phlegm is the clue. *Bronchitis* literally means inflammation of the bronchi, the tubes that connect your windpipe and lungs.

Bronchitis can be either acute or chronic. While both kinds make you feel equally miserable, they progress quite differently. Acute bronchitis usually results from an especially persistent cold or flu virus. It can clear up on its own and shouldn't last more than a week. Chronic bronchitis is usually associated with smoking. It can drag on for months or come and go for years. It's serious enough to require a doctor's care.

With either type of bronchitis, getting all that mucus up and out of your lungs is important because mucus-filled lungs are a potential breeding ground for bacteria that cause pneumonia. The following remedies can help clear your lungs and keep you comfortable while the virus runs its course. If your symptoms persist after 2 days of self-care, see your doctor.

Hit the shower. A comfortably hot shower or bath helps loosen stubborn phlegm. It won't make the virus go away any faster, but it'll sure make you feel better.

Treat your feet. Soak your feet in a hot footbath for 10 minutes. The heat helps draw congestion away from your head, neck, and lungs.

Note: Don't use this remedy if you have diabetes or any condition that affects circulation.

Make a mug of mullein tea. The herb mullein, a member of the snapdragon family, can help rid your lungs of mucus. To make a tea, steep 2 teaspoons of dried mullein leaves in a pot of freshly boiled water for 10 minutes. Strain the tea, then allow it to cool slightly before drinking. Repeat three times a day. You can buy dried mullein leaves in health food stores.

Increase your vitamin C. Research shows that vitamin C reduces the severity of viral infections, including bronchitis. Take 2,000 milligrams a day in supplement form at the first sign of illness, and continue for a few days after you feel better.

Note: Some people develop diarrhea when taking large doses of vitamin C. If this happens to you, cut back your daily dosage to 1,000 milligrams or less until the problem subsides.

Rest your bones. That achy, tired-all-over feeling is your body's way of telling you to slow down so that it can heal itself. Listen to it. Stay home from work if necessary.

Colds

Despite amazing advances in modern medicine, not to mention the more than 800 cold remedies on the market today, scientists have yet to identify a cure for this common malady.

Cold medicines, however, aren't totally useless. They help tame the symptoms. But they do carry a host of side effects, such as drowsiness and dry mouth.

If you want relief without the cost and side effects of over-the-counter drugs, try these natural remedies. (See your doctor if you have a cold with a fever over 101°F for more than a couple of days or if your cough worsens.)

FOLK REMEDY: DOES IT WORK?

Chicken Soup for a Cold

While no one has claimed that chicken soup can cure a cold, it can make you feel better. "Chicken soup is a form of hydrotherapy for your throat," says Angela Stengler, N.D., a naturopathic physician in Oceanside, California. Inhaling the steam from a hot bowl of soup—or sipping any hot liquid—increases bloodflow to the affected area. White blood cells can then get there quickly and start fighting infection faster. "And it increases and loosens mucus flow from your nose," she adds.

Chicken soup can also boost your energy when you're feeling lousy. "If you're sick and not eating, your blood sugar level falls, making you feel worse," Dr. Stengler says. "Food raises your blood sugar level and makes you feel better."

You can fortify your chicken soup with cold-fighting herbs, such as garlic and ginger. "Garlic is antibacterial, antifungal, and antiviral," notes Dr. Stengler, "while ginger calms the stomach and is a decongestant." You can also spice up your soup with hot peppers, which help increase circulation and get those white blood cells moving.

Recommendation: Worth a Try

Start with zinc. Taking zinc gluconate lozenges at the first sign of a cold may reduce the duration of your symptoms. Researchers suspect that zinc works by thwarting viral replication or preventing a virus from entering cells. You can buy zinc gluconate lozenges in health food stores and drugstores.

Try echinacea. Echinacea stimulates disease-fighting white blood cells to fend off cold viruses. The herb is available in a variety of forms in health food stores and some drugstores. Look for capsules that supply 125 milligrams of echinacea extract, standardized to contain 4 percent total echinacosides (the herb's active ingredient).

Note: Don't use echinacea continuously for more than 12 weeks, to give your body a break. If you have an autoimmune disease, such as lupus or multiple sclerosis, don't use echinacea at all. And don't use it if you're allergic to other plants in the daisy family, such as chamomile.

Reach for garlic. Garlic has potent antibiotic and antiviral properties, so taking it in supplement form may minimize cold symptoms. Look for enteric-coated garlic capsules in health food stores. The usual dosage is 300 milligrams three times a day until symptoms subside. Or, if you like yours raw, eat 1½ cloves each day.

Drink a lot. Your body uses up fluids when fighting a cold virus, so staying hydrated is critical. Make sure that you're drinking at least eight 8-ounce glasses of water a day. Steer clear of sweetened fruit juices and sodas. They act as diuretics, flushing water out of your system.

Elevate your head. Propping your head on pillows when you lie down makes breathing easier, especially if you have postnasal drip.

Congestion

You can relieve occasional bouts of congestion on your own. If you frequently feel congested or stuffy and you're not getting better, check in with your doctor. The same advice applies if the congestion is accompanied by green or yellow phlegm, severe headache or facial pain, fever, or persistent cough.

Here's what to do to nip this problem in the bud.

Get steamed. Pour 3 cups of water into a pot and bring it to a simmer. Remove the pot from the stove and set it where you can sit in front of it, such as on your kitchen table. Lean over the pot and drape a towel over your head. (Don't put your face too close to the steam, though, or you may burn yourself.) Inhale the steam for 5 minutes. This should help loosen the mucus in clogged nasal passages.

Mix a scented rub. Camphor, eucalyptus, and menthol are natural decongestants. You can make a rub from any of these essential oils by mixing a couple drops in a handful of corn oil. Put it on your temples, beneath your nose, on your neck—anywhere you can smell it. Essential oils are sold in health food stores and bath-and-beauty shops. If it irritates your skin, don't use it.

Heat up your meals. Hot pepper helps open clogged nasal passages by thinning mucus and making your nose run. Try sprinkling ground red pepper, red-pepper flakes, or hot-pepper sauce on your food.

Make your own nasal spray. A homemade saline solution can clear your nose of irritants such as dust, pollen, and pollution. To make the solution, add ½ teaspoon of salt and a pinch of baking soda to 1 cup of lukewarm water. Spritz the solution into your nose a few times, using a child-sized bulb syringe. Then blow your nose.

Throw the spray away. Over-the-counter nasal sprays and decongestants may provide quick relief, but overuse can cause a rebound effect. In other words, once you stop using them, the stuffiness could come back worse than before. If you use nasal sprays, stop the treatment after 3 days. Don't use decongestants for more than 7 days.

FOLK REMEDY: DOES IT WORK?

Hot Toddy for Congestion

The toddy has a long history of being the best cure for congestion. Basically, it's a hot drink composed of boiling water, a sweetener, and spices, spiked with a shot of liquor.

Does the toddy work? Yes, if you omit the alcohol, says Susan Calvert Finn, R.D., Ph.D., director of nutrition at Roth Laboratories in Columbus, Ohio, and author of *The American Dietetic Association Guide to Women's Nutrition for Healthy Living*. Although liquor can help bring on the virus-fighting sweats, it stresses your immune system. It can also temporarily increase nasal congestion. And alcohol is initially a stimulant—not exactly the gentle treatment you're looking for when you need a long winter's nap.

So mix up a hot toddy without the alcohol to soothe your swollen membranes and help break up mucus. Add a tea bag of chamomile or peppermint leaves to boost the soothing qualities, and be sure to inhale the steam to lubricate your nasal passages.

Recommendation: Worth a Try

Coughing

Coughing clears your airways of mucus, phlegm, and other undesirable matter that you'd much rather be without. Of course, that's hardly comforting when you're hacking away during a meeting, a church service, or your kid's piano recital. At times like these, you just want to get your coughing under control. Here's how.

Have some licorice. The sweet taste of licorice—the herb, not the candy—soothes the throat. And, according to studies, licorice suppresses the cough reflex. To make a tea, add ½ teaspoon of licorice root to a cup of freshly boiled water. Allow to steep for 10 minutes, then strain and allow to cool slightly before drinking.

Note: Don't take licorice more than three times a day or for more than 2 weeks, especially if your blood pressure tends to be high.

Take your thyme. Thyme is a natural antimicrobial and expectorant. It also relaxes airway muscles, which helps stymie a cough. To make a tea, pour ¾ cup of freshly boiled water over 2 teaspoons of fresh thyme leaves or ½ to ¾ teaspoon of dried leaves. (Use medicinal-quality thyme from a health food store, not the thyme in your spice rack.) Cover and steep for 10 minutes, then strain and allow to cool slightly before drinking. Repeat three times a day for up to 3 days.

Drink carrot juice. Put a few drops of vegetable oil in a glass of fresh carrot juice, then take frequent sips throughout the day. Carrots are loaded with vitamin A, which strengthens your respiratory system and can quiet your cough. The vegetable oil coats and soothes your throat.

Ear Infections

Kids may corner the market when it comes to ear infections, but that doesn't mean grown-ups can't get them too.

Many doctors recommend antibiotics for any type of ear infection for two reasons. First, a severe infection, left untreated, can lead to hearing loss. Second, a severe infection could spread to structures close to the ear, causing more serious problems.

So if you suspect that you have an ear infection, see your doctor. Then use these home remedies in conjunction

Unclog Those Ears the Right Way

Earwax traps dirt, dust, and other foreign particles before they travel inside your ear, where they can damage your eardrum, says Jennifer Derebery, M.D., assistant clinical professor of otolaryngology at the University of Southern California and associate of the House Ear Clinic and Institute, both in Los Angeles. But some ears produce too much or unusually hard wax. If it isn't removed, it can cause pain and even temporary hearing loss.

If you have a punctured or perforated eardrum, see your doctor. Otherwise, try this procedure.

1. Using an eyedropper, place a few drops of room-temperature baby oil in your ear. Repeat twice a day for 2 or 3 days. The oil softens and liquefies wax.
2. If the wax doesn't come out on its own, then on the third or fourth day, fill a small bulb syringe with warm water. Pull your ear up and back in the direction of the crown of your head to open up the ear canal. Tilt your head to the side and gently squirt the water into your ear. (You may have to repeat this step a few times.)
3. Once the wax flows out, put an eyedropperful of a solution of half vinegar and half rubbing alcohol into your ear and let it drain out. This dries the ear canal and helps prevent infection.

Under no circumstances should you use cotton swabs or other pointy objects to poke inside your ear, Dr. Derebery cautions. All that does is jam the wax deeper into the ear canal.

with antibiotic treatment to quickly relieve ear pain and discomfort.

Feel the heat. Hold a hot-water bottle, a hot towel, or a heating pad over the affected ear for up to 20 minutes. (If you're using a hot-water bottle or a heating pad, warm it to a comfortably hot temperature and wrap it in a towel before applying it.) The heat stimulates bloodflow, which alleviates pain. It also marshals white blood cells, your body's infection fighters, to the ear area.

Add a little mullein oil. An oil extract made from the herb mullein, a member of the snapdragon family, has potent antibacterial properties. Put a bottle of the oil (sold in health food stores) in a small pan of water and carefully heat it over low heat until it's warm but not hot. Gently shake the bottle, then put a drop or two of the oil on your wrist. If the temperature feels comfortable, use an eyedropper to put a drop of the oil in the affected ear. To coax the drops into your ear, gently pull your ear back and up to straighten the ear canal. Plug the ear's opening with a wad of cotton. Repeat two or three times a day until the infection clears. Don't use this remedy if your eardrum is perforated.

Take a deep breath. The deep-breathing techniques practiced in Qigong, a Chinese healing discipline, may help relieve ear pain. Here's one to try: Imagine that the area from behind your navel to your upper chest is an accordion. Inhale through your nose to fill this area with air and expand the accordion. Then exhale, allowing the air to escape through your lips and collapse the accordion. Continue breathing this way until you feel relaxed and your ear pain subsides. Repeat as needed over a 24-hour period.

Make your own ear drops. A homemade concoction of alcohol and vinegar can help clear up swimmer's ear and keep it from coming back. The alcohol evaporates the water trapped inside your ear, while the vinegar kills the infection-causing bacteria. Combine equal parts rubbing alcohol and distilled white vinegar in a clean eyedropper bottle. Use the eyedropper to put a few drops of the solution in the affected ear. To coax the drops into your ear, gently pull your ear back and up to straighten the ear canal. One application may be all you need to cure swimmer's ear, but it's a good idea to use drops after every swim to prevent future infections. (If you've ever punctured your eardrum, this remedy isn't for you.)

Laryngitis

No one has ever gone mute from laryngitis. The voice usually returns to normal within a few days. But if you have a few things more that you have to say and you just can't wait, try these remedies.

Reach into the candy jar. Sucking on a piece of hard candy can be quite soothing. It increases the production of saliva, which wets your parched voice box.

Make lemon-aid. Squeeze the juice from one or two fresh lemons. Add a tablespoon of honey and a pinch of ground red pepper. Take a sip of this concoction every few hours throughout the day. (If your mouth or stomach is very sensitive, skip this remedy.)

Create a mini-sauna. Bring 3 cups of water to a simmer, then remove the pot from the stove. Add ¼ teaspoon of eucalyptus or peppermint essential oil. Sit or stand so that your face is over the pot. (Don't get too close, though, or you could burn yourself.) Drape a towel over your head and breathe in the steam. Come up for air after 5 minutes.

Rely on water. When you have laryngitis, what feels like phlegm is actually swollen tissues. So repeatedly clearing your throat only makes matters worse. Instead, take frequent sips of water for relief.

Walking Pneumonia: A Misleading Name

Walking pneumonia usually begins as an infection in the upper respiratory tract, often with a sore throat, and progresses to a cough within a few days. Later on, you may develop fatigue, malaise, and a low-grade fever. After a week, it is time to see your doctor. Even though you may not feel all that bad, your sickness will only get worse if you don't determine the cause, says Deirdre O'Connor, N.D., a naturopathic doctor in Mystic, Connecticut.

Even though natural remedies can't cure the problem, they can help keep you from getting it again by keeping your immune system in top shape. Here is what Dr. O'Connor suggests you do.

- Take between 1,000 and 3,000 milligrams of vitamin C a day. Eat plenty of foods that are high in vitamin C, such as broccoli, brussels sprouts, sweet red peppers, sweet potatoes, and citrus fruits.
- Make sure that your daily multivitamin has 15 milligrams of zinc in it. Immune cells can't fight off infection unless they have this mineral. You'll also find zinc in meats, poultry, eggs, dairy products, and oysters.
- Brew an immunity soup. Start with a basic vegetable broth, then toss in sweet red peppers, winter squash, carrots, garlic, onions, and any other colorful vegetables. They contain beta-carotene and other carotenoids that enhance the work of the immune system.
- Cook with lots of garlic and onions. They have antiviral and antibiotic properties to help your immune system fight off both viral and bacterial pneumonia.

Act speechless. Refrain from speaking while you have laryngitis. If you must speak, keep your voice soft and low-pitched, but don't whisper. Whispering actually strains your vocal cords. Likewise, avoid gargling, because it irritates your vocal cords.

Sinus Infections

With each of the 23,000 breaths you take per day, you expose your nose to disease-causing viruses and airborne particles of dust, pollen, and smoke. Sometimes these foreign invaders irritate the mucous membrane that lines your nasal passages. The resulting pain and stuffiness are classic symptoms of a sinus infection, also called sinusitis.

Acute sinusitis usually results from a cold or flu virus. While acute sinusitis makes you feel rotten, it's relatively short-lived. It should clear up in 10 to 14 days. Chronic sinusitis, on the other hand, is milder but more persistent and is usually associated with environmental triggers. Symptoms can linger for months.

No matter which type of sinusitis you may have, you can relieve your symptoms with the following self-care measures. If you don't notice any improvement within 2 weeks, see your doctor.

Give your nose a workout. Using your index fingers, press into the small depression on the outside of each nostril. Hold for 5 seconds, slowly exhaling through your mouth. Then release for 5 seconds, slowly inhaling through your nose. Repeat several times. This exercise should clear congestion and have you breathing better in minutes.

Be a hothead. Applying moist heat improves circulation and delivers vital oxygen and nutrients to your sinuses so they can heal more quickly. Drape a comfortably hot, moist towel directly over your face, covering the area from the middle of your forehead to your upper lip. Leave the towel in place for 5 to 15 minutes. Repeat twice a day.

Raise your legs. Lie on your back with your legs raised against a wall and your buttocks pressed against the wall's base. Stay in this position for 7 to 15 minutes. At first, the pressure in your sinuses will increase. But then it will subside as the mucus loosens up. (Avoid this exercise if you have high blood pressure or glaucoma or are at risk for stroke.)

Drink ginger tea. Because it's so rich in zinc, ginger can help reduce the inflammation and congestion associated with sinusitis. To make a tea, finely chop a ¼-inch slice of fresh ginger and add it to a cup of water in a nonaluminum pot. Cover the pot and let the water boil for 10 to 15 minutes. Strain the tea and allow it to cool slightly before drinking. Repeat as needed.

Note: If you have gallstones, skip this remedy.

Sip with abandon. Drinking plenty of water keeps the nasal passages moist. Aim for at least eight 8-ounce glasses a day.

Humidify your environment. Use a cool-mist humidifier year-round, setting it so that the mist falls close to your face. Be sure to clean the appliance regularly, following the manufacturer's instructions.

Urinary Tract Infections

One in every five women will contract a urinary tract infection sometime in her life. And once you've had one, you're very likely to get more.

Urinary tract infections produce a few telltale symptoms: a frequent, urgent need to urinate; stinging, burning, or pain when urinating; passing just a few drops of urine at a time; and passing blood in the urine. Left untreated, these symptoms usually go away on their own in 3 to 7 days.

Urinary Tract Infections: A Woman's Problem

When it comes to urinary tract infections (UTIs), anatomy rules. A woman's urethra, the tube through which urine flows out of the body, is much shorter than a man's. So any bacteria outside your body can creep up into your bladder much more easily than bacteria can climb the considerably longer male urethra. The bacteria set up shop, and before long, you have a urinary tract infection.

Women also tend to "hold it" longer than men, especially when they are away from home and either don't like the places available to go to the bathroom or have to endure long waits for public restrooms. Putting off urination increases the chances of developing an infection because bacteria aren't getting flushed out as frequently, says Dorothy Barbo, M.D., medical director of the University Center for Women's Health at the University of New Mexico School of Medicine in Albuquerque.

After menopause, women have an added strike against them. As women age, the lining of the urethra becomes thinner, allowing bacteria to ascend into the bladder even more easily. So the older you get, the more vigilant you need to be about preventing UTIs.

Women are more susceptible to urinary tract infections right before menstruation and during menopause, most likely because of hormonal changes. Certain birth control methods also appear to increase risk. Diaphragms, for instance, may kink the urethra, preventing the bladder from emptying completely. And spermicides may change the vaginal flora, causing an overgrowth of *Escherichia coli* bacteria.

If you suspect that you have a urinary tract infection, see your doctor to rule out a more serious problem. She may prescribe antibiotics to kill the bacteria that caused the infection in the first place. In the meantime, these tips can help alleviate your discomfort and prevent future infections.

Order a baking soda cocktail. When you feel a urinary tract infection coming on, add ½ teaspoon of baking soda to 1 cup of water and drink the mixture. The baking soda raises the pH (acid-base balance) of irritating, acidic urine.

Buy berries in a bottle. An as-yet-unidentified substance in cranberry juice prevents bacteria from adhering to the walls of the urethra and bladder. Drink three 8-ounce glasses of cranberry juice cocktail every day until your infection clears. If you don't like cranberry juice, try blueberry juice; it has the same effect.

Flush out bacteria. Drinking water increases urine flow, washing bacteria out of your urinary tract. As a treatment, drink one 8-ounce glass of water every hour for 8 hours.

Sit in a soothing bath. To ease the external burning, take a soak in a bath with essential oils and vinegar. In a small dish, combine 2 tablespoons of honey with the following essential oils, available at health food stores: three drops of sandalwood (an antibacterial), two drops of tea tree (an antiseptic), and one drop of chamomile (an anti-inflammatory). Fill your bathtub halfway with warm or tepid water, then add 2 tablespoons of apple cider vinegar and the honey–essential oil mixture. Sit and soak for 15 to 20 minutes.

Raise your C level. Vitamin C inhibits the growth of bacteria in the urinary tract. Try taking 2,000 milligrams every day for up to 3 days.

Note: Some people develop diarrhea with high doses of

vitamin C. If this happens, reduce your dosage until the problem subsides.

Vaginitis

Vaginitis is known by many names and is caused by many things. But all of the causes produce the same result: burning, itching, discharge, and a whole lot of squirming. The most common form, bacterial vaginosis, occurs when something disturbs the balance among the microorganisms living in the vagina.

Trichomoniasis is the sexually transmitted form of vaginitis. It's caused by a protozoan that gains access to the genitourinary tract. But the best known is the yeast infection, which is caused by an overgrowth of the fungus *Candida albicans* in the vagina.

Vaginitis tends to surface during times of hormonal fluctuation, such as before menstruation and during pregnancy. The risk also rises after menopause, when the vaginal walls become thinner and more vulnerable to infection.

If you experience symptoms of vaginitis, see your doctor. Though vaginitis itself usually isn't serious, it can lead to more serious problems if not properly treated. Your doctor will likely prescribe antibiotics or vaginal cream, which should provide relief in 2 to 3 days. The following remedies can help speed relief of itching and discomfort.

Try the T-treatment. Soak a tea bag in hot water, allow it to cool in the refrigerator, then apply it to the vaginal area. The tannin in the tea can soothe the affected area and relieve itching. (This remedy is intended for external use only.)

Go for the cold. Instead of a tea bag, try laying a clean, cold washcloth against the affected area. The cold causes blood vessels to constrict, which reduces inflammation.

Do a no-soap soak. Sitting in a shallow sitz bath, or even a regular bath, can soothe irritated vaginal tissues. But skip the bubbles or any kind of soap. They leach out your skin's natural oils, which protect against germs.

Eat your yogurt. If you have bacterial vaginosis, eat 8 ounces of yogurt containing live cultures every day to help clear up the infection. The acidophilus bacteria in yogurt helps restore normal bacterial balance in the vagina. Not every yogurt has live cultures, so check the labels.

Revise your toilet procedure. When using the toilet, remember to wipe from front to back. This prevents the transfer of germs from the rectal area to the urethra.

Make a yogurt compress. For yeast infections, put ½ cup of plain yogurt on a clean cloth or towel. Apply the compress to the vaginal area for 15 minutes. Then rinse off the yogurt with warm water and dry the area with a blow-dryer on the warm setting. The yogurt helps relieve itching. (This remedy is for external use only.)

Put out the unwelcome mat. C. *albicans*, often known simply as candida, thrives in a warm, moist environment. To create less hospitable living conditions, wear cotton underwear to stay cool and dry, and sprinkle cornstarch over your groin area to absorb moisture.

Eat carrots. Carrots and other foods rich in beta-carotene may protect against yeast infections by bolstering your immune system.

Turn sour on sweets. C. *albicans* loves sugar. When you eat too much of the sweet stuff, the fungus has a feast. So if you're prone to yeast infections, avoid sugary foods.

Allergy Relief

Allergens are everywhere—from dander on the cat to dust mites on the pillow to certain foods and medicines. No one knows why they rile some people and not others. But genetics seems to play a role. "If one or both of your parents have allergies, then you're much more likely to have allergies too," says Marianne Frieri, M.D., Ph.D., director of the allergy/immunology training program at Nassau County Medical Center and North Shore University Hospital, both on Long Island.

Hormone changes during pregnancy and menstruation heighten some women's sensitivity to allergens.

If you suspect that you have an allergy, see your doctor. "The trouble is, it takes a qualified doctor and testing to identify what it is you're really allergic to," Dr. Frieri says. Only then can you successfully adjust your lifestyle.

For help with particular allergic conditions, here's what to do.

Asthma

Asthma is a chronic condition that affects the bronchi (the tubes that carry air in and out of your lungs), making them prone to mucus buildup and infection. Asthma attacks—which include wheezing, coughing, and gasping for air—are usually triggered by something in the environment, such as pet dander, dust mites, molds, pollens, and cigarette smoke, but they can also be brought on by respiratory infections, stress, anger, laughing, crying, and exercise.

During an asthma attack, the inflamed tissues inside your lungs narrow your airways, which become plugged with excess mucus. As the airways swell, the muscles around them constrict, blocking breathing.

Women who have asthma are more prone to attacks before and during their periods, as hormonal fluctuations stimulate mucus production in the nose, throat, and lungs. Asthma also seems to worsen late in the second trimester of pregnancy. But some women have fewer attacks in the month before the baby is due.

If you have asthma, your allergist may prescribe a bronchodilator inhaler. The medicine in the inhaler opens up bronchial passages, allowing you to breathe more easily. In addition, the following self-care measures can help keep you breathing easy.

In a pinch, quaff coffee. If you feel an asthma attack coming on and you don't have your inhaler with you, drink a cup or two of coffee instead. Caffeine works fairly well as a bronchodilator.

Apply pressure. Make your hands into fists and hold them in front of your chest, thumbs pointing up. Using your thumbs, press along the muscles underneath your collarbone until you feel a knotted, sensitive spot on each side of your chest. Press these points with your thumbs for 2 minutes, hanging your head forward and breathing slowly and deeply as you do.

Exhale longer. Inhale and exhale as you normally do. Then, on the exhalation, continue a bit longer than what feels natural, without forcing out your breath. Practice this yoga breathing technique for 15 minutes twice a day. It may serve as a preventive strategy to reduce the number of asthma attacks you experience.

Pay attention to pills. Certain medications, including aspirin, ibuprofen, and other nonsteroidal anti-inflamma-

Nickel Allergies: A Dime a Dozen

Those beautiful new earrings have left your earlobes inflamed, swollen, scaling, and oozing. You're probably having an allergic reaction to nickel, an ingredient in the metal alloys found in most jewelry.

To soothe and heal your irritated earlobes, apply a milk compress, recommends Hilary Baldwin, M.D., associate professor of dermatology and director of dermatologic surgery at the State University of New York Health Science Center at Brooklyn. Pour whole milk into a bowl and add a few ice cubes. Then dip a soft white cloth into the milk, wring it out, and hold it against your ear for 5 to 15 minutes. Do this several times a day. Milk has anti-inflammatory properties and should help clear up the rash within a matter of days.

Finding earrings that are nickel-free can be a challenge. According to Dr. Baldwin, even those considered "pure" gold contain tiny amounts of nickel. The higher the number of karats, the softer the gold—and the more easily nickel leaches out.

Try wearing earrings made of stainless steel, suggests Dr. Baldwin.

If you absolutely must wear allergy-provoking earrings, reduce your risk of a rash by coating the metal components with clear nail polish. Let the polish dry for 24 hours before putting on the earrings, and reapply it each time you wear the earrings.

tory drugs, can make asthma worse. If you experience more symptoms after starting a new medicine or increasing dosage, tell your doctor.

Supplement your diet. Some vitamins and minerals have been found to lessen asthma symptoms. Check with your doctor before adding these to your treatment plan.

- Magnesium may relax the smooth muscle that lines your airways, minimizing the spasms characteristic of an asthma attack. Nutrition experts recommend 100 to 500 milligrams of magnesium one to three times a day, depending on how much your body can tolerate. Start with the lowest dosage and gradually increase. If you experience symptoms such as gas, cramps, or diarrhea, take less until your symptoms subside. *Note:* If you have heart or kidney problems, consult your doctor before taking magnesium.
- Vitamin C may help reduce your coughing and wheezing. Take 1,000 milligrams four times a day. (Excess vitamin C may cause diarrhea in some people.)
- Quercetin, a bioflavonoid (plant compound), works by inhibiting the mast cells, a component of your immune system that causes allergic reactions by releasing histamine. You can buy quercetin capsules in health food stores. Take 250 milligrams a day.
- Fish oil can help reduce bronchial inflammation. In addition to adding oily fish like salmon and mackerel to your diet, experts recommend taking 240 milligrams of fish oil in capsule form twice a day.
- Evening primrose oil may also help reduce inflammation. Capsules are available in health food stores. Take two 500-milligram capsules three times a day. Stop using them if you experience side effects such as headaches, nausea, or diarrhea.

Eczema

If you have allergies, you may also often have bouts with eczema, a pink, scaly rash that itches intensely. The most common type of eczema is atopic dermatitis, an allergic inflammation of the skin that often affects women who have asthma or hay fever. There's also contact dermatitis, an allergic reaction to an external irritant such as hair coloring or detergent.

While researchers have yet to discover a cure for eczema, doctors suggest these steps for relieving symptoms and minimizing flare-ups.

Change the way you bathe. During an eczema flare-up, bathing once or twice a day can make you feel better. But don't soak in hot water. Instead, use lukewarm water and a mild, nonirritating soap. Stay in the tub until your skin starts to pucker and crinkle, a sign that the skin cells have absorbed water and are hydrated.

Moisturize within 3 minutes. To seal in moisture, apply lotion to your skin while it's still damp—within 3 minutes of your bath or shower. Choose a product with minimal fragrance, color, and additives, all of which can irritate the skin.

Take some skin-friendly supplements. Certain nutrients can quickly end an eczema flare-up. Take them as needed. These are available in health food stores.

- Evening primrose oil contains essential fatty acids, which reduce inflammation. Take two to four 500-milligram capsules three times a day. Stop using them if you experience side effects such as headaches, nausea, or diarrhea.
- Quercetin blocks histamine, the substance released by the skin in response to an allergen. Take two 125-milligram capsules daily.

Feed on fish. If you have frequent eczema flare-ups, you may not be getting enough essential fatty acids in your diet. To increase your intake, eat fish rich in omega-3 and omega-6 fatty acids, such as salmon, mackerel, and herring, three or four times a week.

Give your hands the rubber-glove treatment. Cleaning products, soap and water, and even dust can trigger a flare-up. So slip on cotton glove liners and rubber gloves when washing dishes and housecleaning.

Clean clothes carefully. Use a mild laundry detergent and rinse clothes twice to eliminate detergent residue. And steer clear of scented fabric softeners since the fragrances can irritate your skin.

Food Allergies

When you have a food allergy, your immune system mistakenly identifies certain proteins in foods as a threat to your health. Seafood, especially shellfish, commonly triggers allergic reactions. Wheat, corn, soy, nuts, milk, and eggs (especially the whites) cause their share of misery as well.

If you're allergic to a certain food you've eaten, you'll know—usually within 15 minutes. Your tongue will likely swell or itch, and you'll develop a rash on your skin. Other common symptoms include headache, stomach cramps, extreme flatulence, and diarrhea. Rarely, an allergic reaction may result in anaphylaxis, a potentially life-threatening condition in which blood pressure drops, the throat swells shut, and breathing becomes difficult.

True food allergies are actually quite rare. They affect less than 2 percent of the entire U.S. population. Most women who think they have food allergies more likely have food intolerances.

Allergies Come in Many Guises

Here are places troublesome allergens may show up. Read labels to avoid them.

Corn. Look for buretose, cerulose, dextrin, grits, hydrolyzed vegetable protein, lactic acid, sorbitol, vegetable gum, or vegetable starch. Found in bourbon, breakfast cereals, juice, margarines, marshmallows, oils, snack foods, soft drinks, vinegar, vodka, and wheat-based baked goods.

Cow's milk. Look for calcium caseinate, casein hydrolysate, curds, lactalbumin, lactoglobulin, or whey. Found in baked goods, egg substitute products, hot dogs, lunchmeats, nondairy creamers, snack foods, and soups.

Eggs. Look for albumin, egg powder, egg solids, globulin, ovalbumin, ovomucoid, or ovovitellin. Found in all baked goods, chocolate, coffee, ice cream, marshmallows, meat loaf, noodles, polenta, salad dressings, and wines.

Fish. Look for surimi. Found in imitation fish, sauces, and soup stocks.

Nuts. Look for hydrolyzed protein. Found in cookies and other baked goods, fried foods, gravies, sauces, and vegetable oils.

Soy. Look for hydrolyzed vegetable protein, lecithin, soy flour, textured vegetable protein (TVP), tofu, vegetable gum, vegetable oil, and vegetable starch. Found in breakfast cereals, canned soups, cheese substitutes, condiments, fast-food shakes, fried foods, margarine, meats, miso, tempeh, and veggie burgers.

Wheat. Look for farina, gluten, hydrogenated starch hydrolysates, or semolina. Found in ale, beer, breakfast cereals, canned vegetables, gin, gravies, salad dressings, and whiskey.

For more comprehensive information on specific allergies, write to The Food Allergy Network, 10400 Eaton Place, Suite 107, Fairfax, VA 22030-2208.

If you have a food intolerance, you'll experience some of the same symptoms—namely headache and digestive upset. But a food intolerance is never life threatening. And you may be able to continue enjoying a problem food just by modifying how often you eat it.

Only an allergist can say for sure whether you have a food allergy or a food intolerance. Getting an accurate diagnosis is critical, especially since a true allergy can be life threatening.

If you're diagnosed with a food allergy, your doctor will likely advise you to steer clear of the offending food. These strategies can help you do just that.

Scrutinize labels. Food allergens routinely show up where you least expect them. For example, peanuts—which are responsible for more allergy-related deaths than any other food—go into pastries, breads, and meatballs. Even food additives such as emulsifiers and flavorings may contain peanuts. So before you buy any packaged food or beverage, carefully read the ingredient list.

Be inquisitive. When eating out, find out all you can about a dish before ordering it. Ask the server what ingredients are used and how it is prepared. If the server seems unsure, speak to the chef. Don't be shy—your health is at stake.

Check cosmetics labels. Believe it or not, cosmetics may contain food allergens. Milk, for example, is often used to make lipstick.

•

Hay Fever

Hay fever has the dubious distinction of being the most common of all allergies.

The culprit is the pollen released by ragweed in autumn and by certain grasses and trees in spring and summer. And while the sneezing, runny nose, headache, earache, sore throat, and watery eyes respond well to antihistamines, those medicines can make you tired. For hay fever relief without the drowsiness, try these measures.

Get better with nettle. An herb called stinging nettle can nip hay fever symptoms in the bud. Use freeze-dried nettle (available in health food stores) in capsules or teas. Try a small dose at first since some people have a sensitivity to stinging nettle.

Zero in on C. In large doses, vitamin C acts as an antihistamine, but it doesn't work for everyone. If you want to try it, take 2,000 to 5,000 milligrams a day in divided doses.

Note: Some people develop diarrhea when taking more than 1,000 milligrams of vitamin C per day. If this happens to you, cut back your dosage until the diarrhea subsides.

Be wary of melons. If you are allergic to ragweed, you can get an itchy mouth when eating cantaloupe and other melons. If you're allergic to birch wood, you can get the same reaction when you eat apples or pears or drink chamomile tea. Doctors call this oral allergy syndrome. It isn't serious, but if you're bothered by an itchy mouth, steer clear of offending foods.

Inhalant Allergies

Every day you breathe in as much as 2½ tablespoons of smoke, smog, car exhaust, and assorted other unsavory substances. For most of us, they drift by unnoticed. But if you have an inhalant allergy, certain airborne particles—especially pet dander, dust, and mold—can trigger an immune system response that mimics a respiratory infection.

The usual symptoms include congestion, a runny or itchy nose, sneezing, and red, swollen eyes.

Inhalant allergies may be annoying, but unless you have asthma, they aren't life threatening. Here's what to do to keep symptoms at bay.

Snort saltwater. Add ½ teaspoon of salt and a pinch of baking soda to 1 cup of warm water. Allow the salt and baking soda to dissolve, then put the solution in a squeeze/spray bottle or a medicine dropper. Squirt the solution into one nostril, close the other, and sniff deeply. Switch nostrils and repeat to lubricate your sinuses and prevent sinus infection. You can do this three or four times a day.

Get respite for sore eyes. Run cool water over a clean washcloth. Lay the cloth over your eyes and leave it in place until it feels warm.

Fight fire with fire. Increase your consumption of hot and spicy foods such as ground red pepper, chili peppers, and hot-pepper sauce. The heat loosens mucus.

Venture out after noon. If your allergies are triggered by pollen and molds, stay indoors in the morning, when pollen and mold levels are at their highest.

Clean house. The goal is to get rid of dust mites, the microscopic bugs that feed on bits of shed skin and are well-known allergy aggravators. Their favorite hangout is in mattresses, so encase yours in a plastic cover and wash your bed linens in hot (130°F or warmer) water. And if you can, pull up your carpeting, which harbors dust mites, and live with hardwood, tile, or vinyl floors.

Launder with eucalyptus oil. Australian researchers found that laundering a wool blanket with eucalyptus oil slashed the dust mite population in the blanket by 95 percent. Since eucalyptus oil won't combine with all detergents, you first need to make up a test batch. Mix one part liquid dish detergent concentrate with four parts eucalyptus oil. (If the detergent doesn't dissolve the oil and form a clear solution, try a different brand.) Then stir 1 teaspoon of the detergent-oil mixture into a glass of water. If the oil floats to the top within 10 minutes, it won't work. If it passes these tests, then mix 2½ tablespoons of detergent with 10¼ tablespoons of oil. This is enough for a 20-gallon washing machine. Adjust the mixture proportionally if your machine is bigger or smaller. Eucalyptus oil is very strong, so when you use the mixture, first fill your washing machine with warm water to protect the plastic drum inside, then add the detergent-oil mixture, and last add your bedding. Let everything soak for 30 minutes, then finish the wash cycle.

Good Digestion

Contrary to popular belief, digestive problems are not necessarily caused by something you ate. Some digestive ailments—ulcers, for example—have ties to bacterial and viral infections. Others occur as side effects of medications, including antibiotics and prescription steroids.

"There's also evidence that stress can aggravate conditions such as irritable bowel syndrome and inflammatory bowel disease," says Kim Barrett, Ph.D., professor of medicine at the University of California, San Diego, School of Medicine.

Another mystery is why women seem far more vulnerable to digestive problems than men are. Scientists think that hormonal fluctuations may play a role. "Women experience natural changes in their bowel habits during their monthly cycles, which would suggest some hormonal influence," notes Dr. Barrett.

What can you do to keep your digestive system healthy and minimize illness? First and foremost, build your meals and snacks around high-fiber, low-fat foods. And chew foods thoroughly. Saliva contains enzymes that help break down complex carbohydrates.

Exercise may also help digestion. "If your level of overall fitness improves, your digestive function will improve too," Dr. Barrett says.

Colitis

If you have colitis, which is an inflammation of the colon, a flare-up can cause abdominal pain, bloody stools, and diarrhea, sending you to bed with your misery.

No one seems to know why some people get colitis, but there's some indication that it could be related to stress. (Maybe this is why it's more of a woman's disease.) Medical research indicates that bacterial and parasitic infections such as salmonella can also cause colitis. And temporary colitis can occur after taking certain types of antibiotics.

During flare-ups, you most likely can't avoid taking prescription medicine. But along with it, try these natural strategies. They'll help reduce the symptoms and get you back on your feet faster.

Favor bland fare. Eat plain, low-fat, low-fiber foods such as dry toast, boiled skinless chicken, cooked carrots, and gelatin. These will treat your colon kindly.

Avoid crunchy snacks. Popcorn, nuts, and seeds can aggravate an already angry colon. So steer clear until you're feeling better.

Emphasize fluids. The diarrhea associated with colitis can leave you dehydrated. So drink at least 10 glasses of water or juice a day.

Constipation

By and large, doctors blame constipation on poor nutrition—specifically, too many processed foods and too few fiber-rich ones such as grains, fruits, vegetables, and legumes. Ideally, you should be eating at least 25 grams of fiber a day. Yet most people consume just 12 grams a day on average.

Preventing constipation can be as easy as gradually increasing your fiber intake. Work your way up to at least two servings of whole grains and five servings of fruits and vegetables each day. Some top-notch fiber sources include broccoli (2.3 grams per ½ cup), barley (2.9 grams per ½ cup), and raspberries (8 grams per ½ cup). High-fiber cereals provide even more—up to 11 grams or more per serving.

If you still become constipated from time to time, don't depend on chemically based laxatives to get things moving. These products can lead to a condition called lazy bowel, in which you lose your ability to void naturally.

To restore regularity without risk, try these natural remedies.

Sip apple juice. Sorbitol, a natural sugar in apple juice, acts as a laxative. One glass of juice may be enough to stimulate a balky bowel.

Go with the grain. Mix 1 teaspoon of powdered psyllium seed or whole flaxseed in 1 cup of water or juice. Have this drink with each meal until your symptoms subside. Psyllium seed acts as a natural laxative, while flaxseed increases the bulk and water content of stool. (Because psyllium may inhibit the absorption of drugs, try to take it at least 1 hour after taking other medications.)

Don't skip meals. Eating stimulates food to move through the intestines. Breakfast is especially important because it gets your digestive juices flowing.

Get your fill of water. Constipation can be a sign that you're not drinking enough water. To keep your stools soft, aim for at least eight 8-ounce glasses of water a day.

Hit the bricks. Walking for 15 to 20 minutes a day stimulates bowel function, which supports regularity. Maintain a brisk pace—fast enough that talking is difficult but not impossible.

Diarrhea

According to one study, parents who have young children in day care are 10 to 25 percent more likely to develop diarrhea than parents whose kids stay at home. The reason? Viruses and bacteria, including those that cause diarrhea, easily spread within groups of youngsters. And the children pass the germs on to their moms and dads.

But hand-to-mouth infections aren't the only cause of diarrhea. Loose, watery stools can result from consuming a food or beverage that you're sensitive to or that has spoiled. Caffeine, sorbitol (a sweetener added to diet sodas), antacids, antibiotics, and even stress can also contribute to diarrhea.

See your doctor if your diarrhea doesn't go away within 48 hours or if it's accompanied by other symptoms, such as fever, pain, or blood in the stool.

If your busy life has you on a strict timetable, try these natural remedies to speed relief.

Soothe your intestines with tea. Raspberry leaf contains tannins, substances that reduce intestinal inflammation. To make raspberry leaf tea, pour 1 cup of boiled water over 2 teaspoons of the herb. Steep for 2 to 3 minutes, then strain and allow to cool before drinking. You can buy raspberry leaf in health food stores.

Get better with dried blueberries. Dried blueberries contain inflammation-fighting tannins and pectin, a binding agent that helps solidify loose stools. Thoroughly chew and swallow 3 tablespoons of dried berries.

Let slippery elm soothe you. Slippery elm contains a substance that relieves intestinal irritation. Blend a few spoonfuls of slippery elm bark powder (sold in health food stores) with honey until you can roll the mixture into small balls. Dust the balls with more of the powder. When diarrhea strikes, let one ball slowly dissolve in your mouth. Repeat as necessary. Store leftover balls in a closed container in the refrigerator. (To keep the balls indefinitely, dry them in a very low oven—just the pilot light will work—for a few hours.)

Eat light. Consume only clear liquids such as chicken bouillon, herbal tea, and soft drinks (without artificial sweeteners or caffeine) for the first 24 hours after the onset of diarrhea. Then switch to small meals of bland foods such as bananas, rice, and crackers. Stick with this diet until you've been diarrhea-free for 24 hours, so your digestive tract has a chance to recuperate.

Avoid dairy. Eating dairy products while you have diarrhea can make you feel even worse because you temporarily lose your ability to digest lactose, a sugar in milk.

Don't forget fluids. Your body loses a lot of water when you have diarrhea. So drink at least 10 8-ounce glasses of water a day.

Food Poisoning

Millions of Americans contract some form of food poisoning each year. Sometimes, though rarely, it's fatal. Food poisoning is totally preventable, so get familiar with the following advice.

- Set your refrigerator at 40°F or colder.
- Frequently wash your hands while preparing food, especially after handling raw meat, poultry, or fish and before handling other foods or utensils.
- Thoroughly clean the counter and cutting board after preparing food.
- Put away leftovers immediately (food should not be out for more than 2 hours, less in hot weather).

You'll end up with food poisoning if you consume food tainted with bacteria (such as *Escherichia coli* or salmonella) or a virus. These bugs usually populate raw or undercooked meats, poultry, and seafood; raw eggs; and unpasteurized dairy products and juices.

If your symptoms are extremely severe—you have bloody diarrhea and vomiting that cause dehydration—or they don't subside within 4 days, see a doctor. Usually, though, you can nurse yourself back to health with the following self-care measures.

Defeat dehydration. Mix ½ teaspoon of salt and 3 tablespoons of sugar with 1 quart of water. Drink ½ to 1 cup after each episode of diarrhea or 10 minutes after vomiting. Diarrhea and vomiting rob your body of precious liquids. So, in addition, drink plenty of water.

Be kind to your digestive tract. As your symptoms subside and you regain your appetite, very gradually reintroduce foods into your diet. Begin with broth, then add bland foods.

Endure the diarrhea. Don't take antidiarrheal medications while you have food poisoning. Diarrhea flushes bacteria out of your intestines.

Gastritis

Gastritis is kind of like indigestion gone amok. It's a painful but rarely serious inflammation of the stomach lining.

While certain medications like aspirin and ibuprofen can cause gastritis, bacteria called *Helicobacter pylori* are more often associated with it. Gastritis can either be silent or feel like an ulcer. The symptoms of both gastritis and ulcers are alike: abdominal pain or burning below the breastbone. Only a doctor can determine if you have gastritis or a more serious condition.

Gastritis can attack when it's least expected. When it does, here's what to do.

Choose calcium pills over milk. Milk actually makes gastritis worse by triggering the release of stomach acid.

Avoid the hot stuff. While doctors no longer believe that spicy cuisine contributes to gastritis, patients still complain that it triggers an attack. Try cutting back or eliminating it entirely.

Choose painkillers carefully. Switch from aspirin or ibuprofen to acetaminophen to avoid stomach irritation.

Keep antacids at hand. Antacids almost always work at alleviating pain, so keep them handy in your purse. Don't take more than 16 antacid tablets daily. If your symptoms don't improve in 2 weeks, discontinue use and see your doctor.

Heartburn

Every once in a while, stomach acid defies gravity. Rather than flowing south, it heads north into your esophagus. You feel pressure and a burning sensation beneath your breastbone, along with an acidic taste in your mouth. You have a classic case of heartburn—acid reflux.

While over-the-counter antacids remain the heartburn remedy of choice, you may not want to rely on drugs for relief. Fortunately, you have plenty of natural options.

Keep in mind, however, that many people who think they have heartburn are actually having heart pain. So don't take the symptoms lightly. If they don't go away within a few weeks, see your doctor. If the pain from your chest disperses to your shoulders, back, or neck or if it occurs while you're exercising, go to the emergency room immediately.

Take a feet-first approach. Standing up and moving around while you have heartburn helps clear acid from your esophagus. Avoid bending over or lying down, which can push your stomach acid back up.

Watch the clock. Avoid eating anything less than 2 hours before bedtime.

Skip the after-dinner mints. Mint causes the gastroesophageal sphincter to relax, allowing stomach acid to back up into the esophagus. The same goes for coffee (even decaf) and chocolate.

Delay post-meal workouts. Wait at least an hour after a meal before exercising—all that movement promotes acid reflux.

Irritable Bowel Syndrome

Irritable bowel syndrome (IBS) is sometimes confused with colitis. While the two conditions share many symptoms, they affect the digestive tract quite differently. In colitis, the intestinal lining becomes inflamed and ulcerated. In IBS, the lining twitches, spasms, and cramps uncontrollably.

If you have IBS, you probably experience episodes of abdominal pain, gas, constipation, or diarrhea—or a combination of all four symptoms. Some people's symptoms are so volatile that they alter their daily routines so they're always within range of a toilet.

While IBS can't be cured, you can reduce the frequency and severity of flare-ups with natural remedies. (All remedies mentioned are available in health food stores.) If they don't help, see your doctor.

Counteract pain with cramp bark. The herb cramp bark relaxes the muscular intestinal lining, easing the way for stool to exit the body. During a flare-up, take one to three capsules of cramp bark 15 minutes before each meal. Follow the label instructions for dosage.

Go for the oil. In a German study, 90 percent of people who took peppermint oil and caraway seed oil during a flare-up reported reductions in IBS pain. To try this remedy, add 5 to 10 drops of each oil to 1 cup of warm water. Drink before each meal.

Note: If you're pregnant, avoid caraway seed oil and peppermint oil. They can harm a developing baby when taken in large doses. Also, taking peppermint oil for an extended time can cause serious stomach upset and inflammation.

Take flaxseed by the spoonful. Flaxseed oil is rich in an omega-3 fatty acid with anti-inflammatory properties. Drizzle 2 tablespoons of the oil onto your morning cereal daily. Or take it straight.

Stir up a fiber supplement. Make your own fiber supplement by combining ¼ teaspoon of powdered psyllium seed, ¼ teaspoon of whole flaxseed, and ½ teaspoon of slippery elm bark powder in 1 cup of water. Then squeeze in the juice from a slice or two of lemon. Drink this two or three times a day for up to 4 days. It works to move stool through your intestines.

Profit from pectin. Apple pectin, a granular supplement, is a good source of fiber. Sprinkle it on your food, or dissolve it in liquid and drink it, to supplement your daily fiber intake.

Add spices later. Season your food after it has been cooked. That way, the spices are less likely to irritate your digestive tract.

Lactose Intolerance

If milk doesn't go down as easily as it used to, there's a good reason. As you get older, your intestines produce smaller and smaller amounts of the digestive enzyme lactase.

Lactase is necessary to break down lactose, a natural sugar found in milk and other dairy products. When your lactase levels decrease, you can become lactose intolerant. The symptoms—bloating, cramping, and diarrhea—can appear 15 minutes to several hours after you consume a dairy product.

Here's what you can do to better tolerate lactose intolerance.

Cut your quantity. Researchers at the University of Minnesota at St. Paul found that nearly everyone in a group of lactose-intolerant people could drink *one* 8-ounce glass of 2 percent milk a day without symptoms. By the way, all milk—fat-free, 1 percent, 2 percent, and whole—has the same amount of lactose.

Choose yogurt over milk. Yogurt containing active cultures has less lactose than most other dairy products. Read labels to find a brand with active cultures.

Buy less lactose. Some food manufacturers offer lactose-free and lactose-reduced versions of milk and other dairy products.

Watch for lactose in disguise. Many foods are made with dairy products. Look for milk, cheese, or casein (a protein found in milk) among ingredients listed on canned foods, salad dressings, breads, and candy.

Stretch your legs. Walking for 30 minutes can ease bloating.

Take a load off. For stomach cramps, relaxing is a better remedy than staying active. Soak in a bath, prop up your feet, crawl into bed—whatever makes you feel better.

Nausea and Vomiting

It begins as queasiness, a sickly sensation in the pit of your stomach. Sometimes the sensation passes without incident; other times it crescendos into full-fledged vomiting.

Ironically, as bad as vomiting makes you feel, it's sometimes good for you. Nausea and vomiting are often the result of something bad in your body that your body wants to expel. If this is the case, let your body do its job.

If you continue to feel sick for more than 3 days or experience frequent nausea for no apparent reason or after receiving new medication, see your doctor.

Suck on ginger candy. For any type of nausea, ginger is said to work as well as Dramamine. When you start feeling queasy, suck on crystallized gingerroot candy. It's sold in health food stores and gourmet food shops.

Sip a glass of ginger ale. Ginger ale contains enough real ginger to subdue mild nausea.

FOLK REMEDY: DOES IT WORK?

Cola Syrup for Nausea

If you were a kid during the days when soda fountains were popular, chances are your mom bought you a sweet treat for an aching stomach: cola syrup.

"Cola syrup is thought to calm a queasy stomach because the concentrated sugars help relax the gastrointestinal tract," explains Melanie Cupp, Pharm.D., drug information specialist at the West Virginia University School of Pharmacy in Morgantown. "It can actually calm a queasy stomach within minutes. Pregnant women swear by it for relieving morning sickness."

Cola syrup can be bought without a prescription at your neighborhood pharmacy. Just ask your pharmacist. The syrup will lose its ability to relax the stomach if diluted. For this reason, other liquids should not be consumed for at least 15 minutes after taking a dose. No more than five doses (1 to 2 tablespoons each) should be taken within 1 hour; otherwise, stomach pain and diarrhea may occur, explains Dr. Cupp.

Recommendation: Worth a Try

Keep crackers handy. Nibbling on crackers helps take the edge off nausea. Just stick with small portions.

Get fluids going. If you vomit, don't eat anything for a couple of hours afterward, so your stomach has an opportunity to settle down. Then start sipping fluids such as water, flat soda, sports drinks, and chicken broth.

Stomachache

When a stomachache strikes, you'll experience pain, cramping, and possibly constipation or diarrhea. An upset stomach usually goes away on its own within 24 hours. For faster relief, try these stomach-soothing remedies. (If your symptoms don't subside within a few days or if they are severe and a fever or bloody stool accompanies them, see your doctor to rule out colitis, an ulcer, food poisoning, or other serious stomach conditions.)

Turn to herbs. Drink a cup of chamomile or peppermint tea three or four times a day until you feel better. Both of these herbs gently relieve stomach upset. You can buy herbal teas in health food stores and supermarkets.

Note: Chamomile can cause an allergic reaction, but it's rare. If you are allergic to related plants such as asters, chrysanthemums, and ragweed, take caution when drinking the tea.

If you have stomach cramps, try peppermint oil capsules, which also are available in health food stores. Take one capsule two or three times a day between meals until you feel relief.

Note: During pregnancy, women should never take peppermint because it could harm the fetus.

Eat less more often. Small, frequent meals are easier on your stomach than the standard three squares. So eat mini-meals of bland foods.

Take a breather. When you're stressed, deep breathing can stop your stomach from churning. Sit in a straight-back chair and slowly inhale, feeling your abdomen expand. Then slowly exhale, feeling your diaphragm (the muscle that separates your chest and abdomen) relax.

Hit the spot with heat. Lie down and place a hot-water bottle wrapped in a thin towel across your stomach. The heat can relax a knotted stomach or abdominal muscle and relieve pain.

Slurp soup. Chicken soup is a bland food that helps cleanse the digestive tract and relax stomach cramps.

Sip warm ginger ale. Take frequent small sips. Ginger stimulates the production of saliva, which neutralizes stomach acid.

Chew gum. Like ginger ale, chewing gum gets saliva flowing. Chew for 30 minutes at the onset of an upset stomach or heartburn. Avoid gum with artificial sweeteners, which can have a laxative effect.

Loosen your belt. Clothes that fit tightly around your waist put pressure on your stomach.

FOLK REMEDY: DOES IT WORK?

Milk for Ulcers

It's understandable why people with ulcerated innards historically reached for milk. The high alkalinity of dairy products can be soothing for some people, says Susan Calvert Finn, R.D., Ph.D., director of nutrition at Roth Laboratories in Columbus, Ohio, and author of *The American Dietetic Association Guide to Women's Nutrition for Healthy Living*. Yet, because it's a protein, milk is not easy to digest. In fact, dairy products require high secretions of nothing other than stomach acid.

Recommendation: Forget It

Ulcers

Although ulcers have long had a reputation as a "guy problem," men and women get them just about as frequently. But while men are more likely to develop duodenal ulcers (in the upper segment of the small intestine), women are more susceptible to gastric ulcers (in the stomach).

You've also probably heard that ulcers are caused by acidic foods, excessive alcohol consumption, smoking, or stress—and they are. But research now shows that many ulcers can be linked to the spiral-shaped *Helicobacter pylori* bacterium.

Researchers suspect that *H. pylori* does its damage by penetrating and weakening the digestive tract's protective lining, making it more vulnerable to stomach acids.

If you have an ulcer caused by this bacterium, your doctor will likely put you on a course of antibiotics, along with medications to suppress gastric acid. In 90 percent of cases, *H. pylori* ulcers treated with antibiotics never return.

Not every ulcer results from *H. pylori*, however. Some are due to excessive use of aspirin and other nonsteroidal anti-inflammatory drugs, including ibuprofen.

No matter what the cause of your ulcer, a few simple strategies help control the gnawing, burning pain and quicken the healing process.

Steer clear of caffeine and citrus. While experts no longer believe that specific foods cause ulcers, coffee and citrus fruits and juices are known to worsen ulcer symptoms.

Avoid aspirin and ibuprofen. They're bad news for ulcer-prone stomachs. Instead, take acetaminophen for aches, pains, or headaches.

Drink cabbage juice. Cabbage's anti-ulcer power comes from an amino acid that stimulates the mucous membrane in the stomach to thicken. Deep healing results as the pits in your digestive lining close over.

Drinking about a quart a day for 3 weeks has yielded these heroic results. Fresh is certainly best, but if you don't have a juicer, cabbage juice can be found at health food stores, sometimes under the guise of sauerkraut juice. (Mixing cabbage juice with other vegetable or fruit juices may help improve the taste.) You can also munch on half a head of cabbage throughout the day.

Have a little honey. This golden medicine was specifically prescribed by Middle Eastern and Russian folk healers to cure ulcers long before a bacterium was determined to be the cause. Modern science now qualifies honey's tremendous antibacterial properties, validating yet another bit of folk wisdom.

Get a little culture. Acidophilus and lactobacillus are among the friendly bacteria found in cultured food. The more of these good guys you have populating your stomach lining, the less room there is for *H. pylori* to move in and nibble away at your stomach lining.

If you are already taking antibiotics for *H. pylori*, supplement them with 1 cup of yogurt three or four times daily.

Feed your ulcer fiber. Since ulcer pain can roar back when your stomach growls, stay on a standard feeding schedule. Try to get 35 grams of fiber each day by loading up on fruits, vegetables, and whole grains.

Put some spice in your life. Cayenne pepper can stimulate bloodflow to the stomach, which activates healing. Ingest a small capsule of powdered cayenne pepper. Or sip red-pepper tea made by steeping ¼ teaspoon of cayenne pepper in 1 cup of hot water. You can drink this tea on a daily basis to help prevent the recurrence of ulcers. Modern medicine also has shown that pepper has a mild anesthetic effect.

Your Healthy Heart

Unfortunately, heart disease remains the number-one cause of death among Americans, and among women it's even more prevalent than breast cancer. One in two women will die from heart disease, while one in eight will die from breast cancer, according to Alice H. Lichtenstein, D.Sc., professor of nutrition at the Jean Mayer USDA Human Nutrition Research Center on Aging at Tufts University in Boston.

Thanks to the hormone estrogen, women rarely develop heart disease as early in adulthood as men. Estrogen helps keep women's arteries clear and healthy by regulating the amounts of low-density lipoprotein (LDL) cholesterol, the bad kind that clogs, and high-density lipoprotein (HDL) cholesterol, the good kind that escorts LDL from your body.

Estrogen's protective effects diminish at menopause, however, as the body's production of the hormone declines. At menopause, a woman's risk of heart disease begins to climb, and by the time she reaches age 65, it's about equal to a man's. Despite these odds, women tend to pay less attention to heart health than they should. "Some women simply aren't aware of their risk," Dr. Lichtenstein notes. "Other women are aware, but they're not as concerned about it as they are about breast cancer."

Doctors are eager to spread the word that men and women can do a lot to reduce their chances of getting heart disease in the first place. Here's their best advice for minimizing major risk factors—including angina, high blood pressure, and high cholesterol—and keeping your heart healthy.

Prevention Is So Simple

Some risk factors for heart disease—such as age, race, and family history—you cannot change. That said, there's still plenty you can do to prevent heart disease (and even reverse existing damage).

Snuff the butts. For women, smoking stands head and shoulders above all other risk factors for heart disease. A woman who smokes is two to six times more likely to experience a heart attack than a woman who has never smoked. Almost all women who have heart attacks before age 50 are smokers.

Slim down. Carrying a little extra body fat is okay as long as it's settled on your hips, thighs, and backside. But if you are more than 20 percent above your ideal weight or if fat has taken up residence around your waist, your risk for heart disease edges upward.

To quickly calculate your ideal weight, use this simple formula, known as the body mass index (BMI). Divide your weight (in pounds) by your height (in inches) squared. Multiply the resulting number by 705 to get your BMI.

A person who weighs 145 pounds and is 5 feet, 4 inches tall (64 inches), for example, would divide 145 by 4,096 (height in inches squared) to get 0.0354. Then that figure would be multiplied by 705. The answer rounds up to 25 and represents the person's BMI.

Doctors say that a healthy BMI is somewhere between 19 and 24. One large-scale study points to a BMI below 21 as ideal for preventing heart disease.

Be frugal with fat. Saturated dietary fat accelerates the progression of heart disease. Doctors recommend limiting your total daily fat intake to 30 percent of calories, with no more than 7 percent of those calories coming from saturated fat. To help achieve this without doing a lot of arithmetic, limit yourself to no more than 6 ounces of lean meat, fish, or poultry a day and use skim and low-fat dairy products.

Use olive oil in place of other fats. Olive oil consists mostly of monounsaturated fatty acids, which have been shown to lower LDL cholesterol levels while raising HDL levels. But don't go overboard; oil is still 100 percent fat.

Fill up with fiber. By substituting high-fiber foods for high-fat ones, you'll decrease your LDL cholesterol. Add oat bran, oatmeal, barley, and beans to your menus for a good dose of soluble fiber, the type that researchers say is especially effective.

Make produce your pal. Build your meals around a variety of foods, including plenty of antioxidant-rich fruits and vegetables. Antioxidants—vitamins C and E and beta-carotene—neutralize highly destructive molecules called free radicals. In this way, the nutrients defend artery walls against the damage that triggers plaque accumulation. Eat at least five servings a day of antioxidant-rich fruits and vegetables, including broccoli, carrots, collard greens, Swiss chard, citrus fruits, papaya, and cantaloupe.

Include tomatoes too. Tomatoes are the best source of lycopene, a compound that appears to protect against heart disease. Just ½ cup of tomato sauce supplies 22 milligrams, ¾ cup of tomato juice has 20 milligrams, and ½ cup of chopped fresh tomatoes supplies 8 milligrams.

Give garlic the green light. Garlic contains allicin, a compound that appears to lower cholesterol and blood pressure. Eat one clove a day, using chopped, fresh garlic to flavor salads and cooked dishes.

Sip a little wine (or grape juice). Compounds known as flavonoids may prevent LDL cholesterol from sticking to artery walls and may stop blood platelets from clumping together and forming dangerous clots. Flavonoids are found in abundance in red wine and grape juice. Other sources include onions, apples, broccoli, and tea. If you choose to drink red wine, keep in mind that studies have shown moderate alcohol consumption—just one drink a day—increases breast cancer risk by 30 to 40 percent. If you have a family history of breast cancer, restrict yourself to two or three drinks a week. A drink equals 5 ounces of wine.

Invest in supplemental insurance. Even if you eat healthfully, you may not get enough of certain nutrients to protect against heart disease. A multivitamin/mineral supplement can cover any deficit. Make sure that your multivitamin contains vitamin B_6, vitamin B_{12}, and folate. These nutrients help prevent the chemical changes that lead to atherosclerosis (hardening and clogging of the arteries).

Do some legwork. Make sure you do a minimum of 30 minutes of heart-pumping aerobic activity (such as brisk walking, running, or cycling) three or four times a week. Aerobic exercise strengthens and tones your heart muscle, so your heart pumps more blood with each beat. And it reduces the stickiness of platelets, making them less likely to form clots.

Control diabetes. Diabetes can increase your risk for heart disease fourfold. If you have diabetes, work with your doctor to develop a diet, exercise, and weight-loss program geared toward monitoring and managing your blood sugar levels.

Angina

The recurring pressure in your chest has you wondering whether you're experiencing the first signs of heart trouble. You're wise to wonder, because angina is a warning sign that should never be ignored.

Angina occurs when your heart isn't getting enough oxygen-rich blood. The resulting pain—usually in your chest but sometimes in your jaw or arm—subsides once your heart's oxygen needs are met.

As it turns out, not everyone who has angina eventually experiences a heart attack (when bloodflow to the heart becomes completely blocked). In fact, angina seems less likely to lead to heart attacks in women than in men.

If you have angina, your doctor will most likely prescribe nitroglycerin, a medication that dilates the heart's arteries. Follow her instructions carefully when using this medication. In addition, try the following strategies to minimize angina pain and discourage future attacks.

Stop what you are doing. When you feel an angina attack coming on, sit down and rest. If you have clogged arteries, this reduces the workload on your heart and alleviates pain.

Thwart attacks with hawthorn. Research has shown that the herb hawthorn contains substances that open arteries and improve bloodflow to the heart. Naturopathic doctors recommend taking 240 to 480 milligrams of standardized hawthorn extract each day. While hawthorn is natural, it is a powerful medicine, so do not take it without first discussing it with your doctor.

High Blood Pressure

One out of every four people between the ages of 35 and 55—and one of every two over age 55—has high blood pressure. Most don't even know it.

Doctors define high blood pressure as a consistent reading of 140/90 mm Hg (millimeters of mercury) or higher. A reading that is 120/80 is considered ideal.

High blood pressure is as mysterious as it is silent. Scientists don't know why some of us get high blood pressure, but they do know that certain factors contribute to a woman's vulnerability.

- Ethnic background—African-American, Puerto Rican, Cuban, or Mexican
- Overweight
- Birth control pills
- Stress
- Diabetes or a disease that affects the kidneys, adrenal glands, or other glands

High blood pressure is potentially dangerous because it stresses the arteries, putting you at risk for heart attack and stroke. Left untreated, it can also lead to kidney failure.

Medication can help control high blood pressure, helping to prevent its potential damage. If you can't get it under control using natural methods, your doctor may prescribe medication. But nondrug options like the following can knock points off your reading too. (If you are already taking blood pressure medication, be sure to consult your doctor before making any changes in your dosage.)

Savor the "stinking rose." Studies show that allicin, the compound in garlic that helps lower cholesterol, reduces blood pressure as well. The suggested intake is one clove per day.

Tap the power of potassium. In one study, a daily 3,120-milligram dose of potassium slashed an average of seven points from participants' systolic blood pressures (the top number in a reading). Their diastolic pressures (the bottom number) also dropped an average of two points. Good food sources of potassium include baked potatoes, cantaloupe,

Low Blood Pressure: Women's Luck?

Thanks to the female hormone estrogen, women often have lower blood pressure readings than men. It's only when your typical reading drops significantly that something might be wrong.

"Low blood pressure puts you at lower risk for cardiovascular disease, stroke, and kidney disease. It's usually something to be glad about," says Clarita E. Herrera, M.D., clinical instructor in primary care at the New York Medical College in Valhalla, New York, and attending physician at Lenox Hill Hospital in New York City.

The only problem with low blood pressure (hypotension) is that it can make you lightheaded when you move your body quickly. The key is to be aware of this and train yourself to move mindfully, Dr. Herrera says. When you're getting out of bed, for example, pause in a seated position and take a few deep breaths.

Also keep in mind that as levels of protective estrogen decline during menopause, your blood pressure could start going up (as does your risk for heart disease). Be sure to have it checked regularly.

and spinach. Other potassium-rich foods include bananas, beans, honeydew melon, orange juice, prunes, and raisins. Aim for an intake of 2,000 to 4,000 milligrams a day.

Count up calcium. At least two studies have found that moms-to-be who take supplemental calcium reduce their chances of developing pregnancy-related high blood pressure. If you're pregnant or nursing, you need 1,200 to 1,500 milligrams of calcium a day.

Check out coenzyme Q_{10} and l-carnitine. When taken together, coenzyme Q_{10} (an antioxidant) and l-carnitine (an amino acid) may help lower blood pressure and strengthen heart muscle contractions. Both supplements are sold in health food stores.

Salt sensibly. Salt is not the cardiovascular villain it was once thought to be. In fact, some research suggests that consuming up to 4,000 milligrams of sodium a day won't necessarily raise your blood pressure, as long as you're also taking in enough magnesium and potassium. Still, you're wise to use salt judiciously. Limit yourself to 1 teaspoon (2,000 milligrams) a day.

Crunch celery. Thanks to its mild diuretic properties, celery may help lower blood pressure by reducing the amount of fluid in the bloodstream. Eat at least four stalks a day.

High Cholesterol

With all we've heard about the dangers of cholesterol, you'd think it's something we could gladly do without. The truth is that we can't live without cholesterol. It's only when levels get too high that we have to do something about it.

What constitutes "high" is also up for debate. Some researchers say that to be completely on the safe side, your total cholesterol reading should be under 150 mg/dl (milligrams per deciliter), which is difficult for some people to achieve. More commonly, we're told that a total reading of 240 is the safe limit.

Recently, researchers have been finding that it's not total cholesterol at all but the ratio between good HDL and bad LDL that's the leading indicator. The total doesn't matter as long as your LDL is no higher than 130 and your HDL is 45 or higher. And the higher your HDL, the better.

This means that if your total comes out on the high side, you don't need to panic. Ask your doctor to take readings for HDL and LDL. If it still doesn't look good, practice the prevention techniques mentioned above. Plus, you can try the following home remedies that studies have shown can help reduce cholesterol.

Befriend fenugreek. In one study, participants who consumed ¾ cup of the herb fenugreek every day for 20 days cut their LDL levels by one-third. (Their HDL levels stayed the same.) Eat 1 to 2 tablespoons of ground fenugreek seeds three or four times a day. If you don't like the taste of the seeds, you can take one or two 580-milligram capsules three or four times a day. Both ground seeds and capsules are sold in most health food stores.

Try turmeric. Turmeric, a staple of Indian cuisine, enhances the body's ability to process cholesterol. Sprinkle the ground herb on poultry, fish, and beans. Or take 150 milligrams in capsule form (available in most health food stores) three times a day.

Make it hot, hot, hot. Hot peppers contain capsaicin, an oil that can keep LDL cholesterol from sticking to artery walls.

Go fishin'. Certain species of fish—including mackerel, salmon, and tuna—are rich in omega-3 fatty acids. Omega-3s may lower heart-harming LDL cholesterol while sustaining heart-healthy HDL. Eat at least one 3-ounce serving of fish rich in omega-3s per week.

Get the flax. Studies have shown that flaxseed lowers LDL while preserving HDL, probably because of its high fiber content. Look for ground flaxseed in health food stores. Sprinkle a tablespoon or more on hot or cold cereal, soup, or yogurt.

Consider C. In one study, people with low vitamin C levels who took 1,000 milligrams of the nutrient every day for 8 months raised their HDL readings by 7 percent, on average.

Pain, Pain, Gone Away

This may come as little comfort when you slip a disk moving the sofa or break a bone running down the steps, but pain is good. Imagine what would happen if you kept running on a broken foot!

Pain comes in two varieties. Acute pain, the kind you get when you bang your knee, comes on suddenly and goes away when the injury is gone. All of us have had it, and we're sure to have it again. It can last for anywhere from a few minutes to a few weeks. A little rest, maybe some ice at first or heat later, and over-the-counter pain relievers are usually enough to get you through it.

The other kind of pain, chronic pain, is more insidious. Some injuries and diseases create pain that lingers on and off for months and sometimes years. It's estimated that more than 67 million people in the United States experience chronic pain.

In this chapter, you'll find natural relief for some of the most common causes of acute and chronic pain. If you have already been diagnosed with a problem and are taking medication for it, do not discontinue your medication without consulting your doctor. If you have pain that's associated with a disease such as lupus or arthritis or if you have unexplained or unbearable pain, see your doctor to find out the cause, cautions Margaret Caudill, M.D., Ph.D., codirector of the department of pain medicine at Dartmouth Hitchcock Clinic in Manchester, New Hampshire, and author of *Managing Pain Before It Manages You.*

Arthritis

If you're over age 45, it's likely that you've already experienced arthritis pain. If not, you surely will by the time you retire, even if it's just a twinge in the knee.

But arthritis isn't just the purview of the aging. In one survey of 24,000 women, nearly 9 percent of those between ages 15 and 44 said that they had arthritis pain.

Researchers have identified more than 100 forms of arthritis. The two most common—and the ones that affect women the most—are osteoarthritis and rheumatoid arthritis.

Osteoarthritis is caused by the gradual breakdown of cartilage, the soft, spongy material that cushions joints. It can also result from injury— that skating accident you had as a kid can show up decades later as arthritis. Overweight is a factor too.

Rheumatoid arthritis is considered a younger person's pain. It affects mostly women in their thirties, forties, and fifties. Medically speaking, it's classified as an autoimmune disease. In other words, the body's immune system turns on itself—in this case causing the synovial membrane, which lubricates each joint, to become inflamed.

For either type of arthritis, many doctors recommend nonsteroidal anti-inflammatory drugs to minimize pain, swelling, and stiffness. The following nondrug remedies can also ease discomfort and improve joint mobility.

Give peas a chance. Wrap a bag of frozen peas in a towel and apply it to the swollen joint for 10 to 15 minutes, two or three times a day. The cold reduces inflammation.

Create a rice pack. To warm painful, stiff joints, fill a soft white tube sock with 5 to 8 inches of uncooked rice. Knot the sock, or tie it shut with string. Heat it in the microwave for 2 minutes, then check the temperature before applying it to the affected joint. If you can comfortably hold the sock, it's not too hot. Rest the pack on the affected area and leave it in place until it cools down. The heat increases blood circulation, which in turn helps loosen and soothe the area.

Reach for the chile. If you have osteoarthritis, try an over-the-counter cream made with capsaicin (a chile pepper extract), such as Capzasin or Arthricare. It depletes a chemical in the nerves, called substance P, that sends pain messages to the brain.

Check out curcumin. For rheumatoid arthritis, take 400 milligrams of curcumin three times a day until the flare-up subsides. Curcumin, the yellow pigment in turmeric, can relieve swelling and improve joint mobility. Curcumin capsules are available in health food stores.

Eat your fish. Certain species of fish, including Atlantic herring and Atlantic salmon, contain omega-3 fatty acids, which have been shown to reduce the inflammation of rheumatoid arthritis. Eat at least one 3-ounce serving of a fish rich in omega-3s each day.

Keep joints moving. While it may seem impossible when you're hurting, exercise can actually reduce pain. Regular low-impact aerobic exercise, such as swimming or riding an exercise bicycle, increases the circulation of fluid around joints and strengthens the muscles that support joints. Avoid exercise if your joints are red, hot, and swollen.

Back Pain

It's almost as common as the common cold, but back pain lingers much longer. In fact, it's responsible for about six million doctor visits a year, many of them from women who spend all day sitting in front of computers.

Most back pain goes away on its own within a few days to a week. But if you don't want to wait it out, these self-care measures can help. If these remedies don't help or if the pain is so great that you can't tolerate it, see your doctor.

Hold it right there. When back pain strikes, stop what you're doing. The pain is your body's way of telling you that you're doing something the wrong way. Try to figure out what's wrong, and make adjustments. Perhaps you can then continue the activity in comfort.

Get help from heat. For back pain caused by a muscle spasm, soak a washcloth in comfortably hot water and place it over the affected area. Resoak the cloth every 3 minutes or so to keep it warm. Continue the applications for up to 30 minutes.

Try ice. To relieve a back injury within the first 24 hours, apply a towel-wrapped ice pack to the affected area for 5 to 10 minutes. Repeat every hour.

Take it lying down. For lower-back pain, lie on the floor with a pillow positioned under your knees so that they bend slightly. This rests your iliopsoas muscles, which extend from your lower back around either side of your body to the thighbone.

Stop pain by stretching. Stop pain before it starts, by relieving tightness and stiffness in your back. Stand in front of a table and bend forward so that you can rest your torso on the table. Your torso should form a 90-degree angle with your thighs. Extend your arms in front of you, then breathe slowly as you bend your knees slightly. Hold for 2 minutes, then brace yourself with your arms and stand up straight.

Move soon. Don't let an aching back keep you in bed for more than 2 days. After 48 hours of bed rest, your circulation slows down, your muscles and joints stiffen, and your back pain gets worse.

Chronic Pain

You may or may not know what causes it. But it doesn't really matter—all you know is that it doesn't go away. Chronic pain is debilitating, and it can affect more than your health. It can cause a dramatic change in your lifestyle and in your relationships with family and friends. But pain doesn't have to be a life sentence.

To control chronic pain, you must deplete the pain-intensifying hormones. One way to accomplish this is through relaxation. Researchers have found that when you're in a relaxed state, pain-intensifying hormones dissipate. Try the following relaxation techniques to ease your chronic pain.

Use your breath. Deep breathing can derail stress, which in turn minimizes pain. Sit in a comfortable chair and place one hand on your chest and one hand on your stomach. Inhale. If the hand on your chest rises more than the hand on your stomach, you're breathing too shallowly. Breathe in deeply again, this time focusing on moving the hand on your stomach, not your chest. Practice deep breathing in this way for about 2 minutes three times a day.

Master meditation. Meditating for 5 to 10 minutes a day can help provide significant relief because it changes your perception of physical pain.

The 10 Best Hemorrhoid Cures

1. To soothe pain and swelling, put a wet washcloth inside a plastic bag and then into the freezer until it freezes. Take the washcloth out of the bag and apply it to the anal area for 10 minutes. Cold makes blood vessels constrict.
2. To relieve itching, apply an over-the-counter hemorrhoidal cream or ointment that contains a numbing medicine such as pramoxine 1% (like Anusol and Hemorid).
3. To reduce inflammation, apply 1 percent hydrocortisone cream or ointment twice a day. Use after a bowel movement or a bath.
4. Soak a cloth in witch hazel and apply to the anal area for 10 minutes.
5. Sit in a bathtub of comfortably hot water for 10 to 15 minutes three times a day. Draw your knees toward your chest so that the water can reach the anal area.
6. If you have external hemorrhoids, use a cotton ball to dab them with an antifungal powder or cornstarch two or three times a day to keep them dry.
7. Avoid constipation. Drink plenty of water and eat high-fiber foods. You can also use a fiber supplement to keep stools soft and regular.
8. Switch to toilet tissue that has added moisturizers.
9. If you can stand instead of sit, do so. Sitting for long periods can aggravate hemorrhoids.
10. Learn to sleep on your side. Lying on your back places your hemorrhoids below the level of your heart. Consequently, blood flows to that area, which increases swelling.

To meditate, sit in a comfortable position on the floor with your back against a wall or in a chair with your feet on the floor and your hands resting on your thighs. Breathe in slowly and deeply for five counts, then exhale slowly for five counts. Close your eyes and concentrate on a soothing, peaceful activity or place where you feel safe and calm.

Relax to music. Listening to music that relaxes or cheers you can help relieve pain.

Stay active. Exercise stimulates the release of endorphins, which raise your pain threshold and produce a sense of well-being. Aim for 20 to 30 minutes of aerobic activity six times a week. (If your pain gets worse, consult your doctor.)

Fibromyalgia

Doctors describe fibromyalgia as a pain syndrome. What hurts are the fibrous tissues of the body: muscles, ligaments, tendons, and fasciae (sheets of connective tissue). Fibromyalgia makes certain points on your body exquisitely sensitive to touch. These tender spots often include the inside edges of the shoulder blades, the base of the head, the outer forearms just below the elbows, and the insides of the knees.

If you have fibromyalgia, use the following strategies to help you feel better, reduce your soreness, and regain your energy.

Take to your tub. Heat relieves fibromyalgia pain. Draw a comfortably hot bath, then climb in for a long soak.

Modify your breathing. A technique called diaphragmatic breathing relaxes tight muscles and improves circulation. Allow the area below your rib cage to expand as you inhale and contract as you exhale. Continue for 5 minutes, doing eight breath cycles per minute.

Stretch to soothe. Fibromyalgia pain causes muscles to tighten. Stretching loosens stiff, sore muscles and makes you feel better.

Think progressively. By using a technique called progressive muscle relaxation, you can relieve some of the tightness associated with fibromyalgia. Begin by gently clenching your fists until you feel the muscles tensing. Hold for 3 seconds, then release. Repeat, working your muscles in the following sequence: arms, shoulders, neck, face, abdomen, lower back, buttocks, thighs, calves, and feet. Repeat twice a day.

Make time for exercise. Even though you hurt, exercise can do you a world of good. Begin with a brisk walk for 5 minutes three times a week, then gradually work your way up to 20 minutes three times a week.

Take a one-two punch. In one study, people with fibromyalgia who took magnesium and malic acid (found in apples) experienced reductions in muscle pain and tenderness. Begin by taking 150 milligrams of magnesium and 600 milligrams of malic acid twice daily for 1 to 2 weeks. Then gradually increase your dosage every 2 to 3 days until you reach 300 milligrams of magnesium and 1,200 milligrams of malic acid twice daily. You can buy combination magnesium/malic acid supplements in some drugstores and health food stores.

Note: If you have heart or kidney problems, check with your doctor before taking magnesium supplements.

Kidney Stones

Some say that the agony caused by kidney stones is equaled only by childbirth. Since stones are much more common among men than women, maybe they're nature's way of evening the score.

The primary symptom of a kidney stone is excruciating

pain in the lower back or abdomen. You may have the urge to urinate more often and experience a burning sensation when you do go. You may notice blood in your urine. You may also feel nauseated, and you may vomit.

Sometimes kidney stones create an obstruction in the kidney or ureter. They can also cause infections that, if left untreated, can do irreparable damage to the kidneys.

Once you've developed a kidney stone, only passing it will bring relief. Here's what you can do to flush that painful pebble out of your system and discourage future formations. (You should seek a doctor's help once you've passed the stone or if the pain is unbearable.)

Drink lots of water. Drink at least eight 8-ounce glasses of water every day. All that fluid dilutes the chemicals in your urine so that calcium and oxalate—the two main components of most kidney stones—can't get together.

Get lots of citrus. Beverages rich in citric acid, such as orange juice and lemonade, inhibit calcium stone formation. Drink ¾ cup of orange juice with each meal or 1¼ cups of lemonade twice a day.

Steer clear of stone formers. Avoid foods that contain stone-forming oxalate, including beans, beets, peanuts, and spinach.

Migraines

A headache is to a migraine what a bicycle is to a tank. And if you've never had one, it's hard to imagine how intensely painful a migraine can be. It's not uncommon for a migraine to drive a person to bed for days in a dark room. Migraines can sometimes be so severe that they cause nausea, vomiting, weakness, and sensitivity to light.

For about 5 to 10 percent of people, a migraine announces its pending arrival with an aura, a visual disturbance characterized by brightly colored lines, flashes of

Migraines More Common in Women

You can thank Mother Nature for the fact that migraines are more common in women than in men. She's the one who provides the estrogen that feeds migraines, the mother of all headaches.

Before puberty, girls and boys get migraines at about the same ratio. But once those hormones kick in, it's a different story. Then the female rate jumps to four times that of males, says Patricia Solbach, Ph.D., director of the Center for Clinical Research at the Menninger Clinic in Topeka, Kansas.

The odds decrease once again as women approach menopause. When menstruation ceases and hormone levels become steadier, migraines usually occur less frequently and can even go away altogether.

A word of caution: If you have migraines and opt for hormone-replacement therapy, your migraines might come back.

light, dots, or spots. The pain itself can last anywhere from 4 hours to 3 days.

Once a migraine gets a foothold, it doesn't want to leave. The following measures can provide some relief and, even better, reduce the frequency and severity of recurrences.

Take a whiff of apple. In one study of people with migraines, the scent of green apples made their migraine pain fade. The reason why is unclear.

Freeze the pain. Cold helps constrict expanded blood vessels and block pain messages to your brain. Wrap ice or an ice pack in a towel and apply for 10 minutes to the area of your head that hurts.

Consider a coffee cure. Like ice, the caffeine in coffee constricts expanded blood vessels in the brain. But limit yourself to one 5-ounce serving (about ⅔ cup), which contains about 100 milligrams of caffeine. Too much coffee can aggravate a migraine.

Mind your magnesium. Italian researchers have found that people who get migraines tend to have lower blood levels of magnesium than people who don't. Good food sources of the mineral include green leafy vegetables, legumes, seafood, and nuts.

Steer clear of trigger foods. You can minimize the frequency and severity of migraines just by avoiding the foods known to cause them. The most common offenders are anything that has been aged, fermented, marinated, or pickled, such as aged cheese, red wine, and pickled herring. Also bypass any foods that contain monosodium glutamate (MSG), nitrates, or nitrites, such as canned soups and lunchmeats.

Neck Pain

Imagine balancing a bowling ball on a pencil. Tough job, wouldn't you say? Now you have some idea what the human neck is up against, trying to support a 14-pound head.

While everyone gets neck pain from time to time, a pain in the neck doesn't have to be a pain in the neck. Here's what you can do to get rid of it.

Go ice and easy. Wrap ice or an ice pack in a washcloth and apply it to your neck for 15 to 20 minutes. The cold relieves stiffness and discomfort.

Stay warm. If your neck pain doesn't respond to cold, try heat instead. Apply a heating pad set on low or medium for up to 20 minutes.

Take a look around. Turn your head all the way to one side. Bring it back to center so that you're looking straight

Give Your Back a Break

Whether It's a heavy handbag hanging off one shoulder or a child resting on one hip, women have a habit of letting one side of their bodies carry all their burdens, says Lois Buschbacher, M.D., a physiatrist in Indianapolis.

When you hoist a heavy purse on your shoulder, you automatically lift the weight-bearing shoulder, causing your neck muscles to cramp and spasm, which leads to neck, shoulder, and back pain.

To avoid strain, carry everything—purses, boxes, bags, children—close to the center of your body. And trade in your shoulder bag for a backpack purse.

Here are two exercises recommended by Dr. Buschbacher to make your neck and shoulder muscles stronger and more flexible.

- While sitting or standing, roll both shoulders forward at the same time, then up and back, and then down to complete a circle. Repeat 10 times, then reverse direction.
- While sitting or standing straight, draw your shoulders back together, with your elbows back and inward. Repeat 10 times.

ahead. Repeat to the other side. Then look down at the floor, raise your head to center, look up at the ceiling, and lower your head to center.

Wear sensible shoes. High heels knock your spine out of alignment, which makes your neck jut forward. So wear flats or low-heeled shoes.

Give your handbag the ol' heave-ho. Slinging a heavy purse over one shoulder strains your neck as well as your back and shoulders. Instead, wear a fanny pack or backpack.

Raynaud's Disease

Cold fingers and toes are to be expected in wintertime. But for people with Raynaud's disease, painfully frigid digits occur year-round. A glitch in the circulatory system causes tiny blood vessels in the fingers and toes to spasm in response to cold. With bloodflow cut off, the fingers and toes become so cold that they ache. They also change color: first white, then blue, then back to red once they warm up.

Doctors sometimes recommend surgery to correct extreme cases of Raynaud's. Before you go that route, try these self-care measures to minimize your discomfort.

Relax in a scented bath. Sitting in a warm (not hot) bath helps increase circulation to the extremities. Mix 1 teaspoon of combined essential oils such as cypress, savory, birch, and rosemary with 1 cup of milk and add to the bathwater. Cypress oil may help the circulatory system, savory serves as an external stimulant, and birch and rosemary may soothe muscular pains.

Put up your dukes. If Raynaud's strikes you when you're walking from one heat zone to another, ball your hands into loose fists. Give your body a few minutes to adjust to the temperature change before releasing your fists.

Make a beeline for E. To improve circulation, take between 400 and 1,200 international units of vitamin E a day.

Can caffeine. Whether from coffee, tea, cola, or over-the-counter medication, caffeine constricts blood vessels and aggravates Raynaud's.

Retrain your cold response. This technique can help either your hands or feet readapt to cold, reducing a Raynaud's reaction. Fill two buckets or plastic foam coolers with 100°F water. Place one container in a cold area—on an outside patio, for example—and the other in a warm room. Wearing lightweight clothes, immerse your hands in the indoor water for 2 to 5 minutes. Wrap your hands in a towel, go outside, unwrap your hands, and immerse them in the outdoor water for 10 minutes. Go back inside and immerse your hands in the indoor water for 2 to 5 minutes. Repeat six or seven times every other day.

This procedure, called the submersion technique, trains your blood vessels to dilate rather than constrict in response to cold.

Repetitive Strain Injury

It happens to typists, cashiers, and even grandmothers who spend their days knitting. If you do anything that involves steadily moving your hands, you are at risk for repetitive strain injury.

The most common repetitive strain injury is carpal tunnel syndrome, which makes your hand, wrist, arm, and elbow muscles feel achy and sore. The median nerve, which runs through the bony carpal tunnel in your wrist, becomes compressed by swollen tendons.

Repetitive strain injury can also affect your neck and shoulders. And it may be accompanied by other symptoms, including tingling, numbness, decreased dexterity, and fatigue.

Experts agree that for repetitive strain injury, prevention is the best medicine. That means scrutinizing your lifestyle and work style to identify and change those practices that may be putting you at risk. Start with the following strategies.

- Rearrange your work areas at home and on the job to reduce repetitive reaching.

- Alternate tasks whenever possible to avoid sequences of activities that use the same muscles and tendons.
- Choose tools that fit your hands if you're a woman. Often, tools are designed for a man's larger hands.
- If you sit for long periods of time, make sure that you have a chair that is properly proportioned for your body.
- If your job requires moderate to heavy phone use, wear a headset.

If, despite your best efforts at prevention, you suspect that you have a repetitive strain injury, don't ignore it. Schedule an appointment with your doctor. Then try the following tips to help manage your pain.

Give yourself a break. If you're involved in a repetitive activity, take a break every 20 to 30 minutes. Roll your shoulders, stretch your muscles, and massage the sore areas to stimulate circulation.

Soothe with a scented self-massage. Massage an herbal oil onto the sore area. Look for a product that contains either Roman chamomile (not German chamomile) essential oil or rosemary and ginger essential oils. All of these oils have anti-inflammatory properties. They're sold in health food stores and some bath-and-beauty shops.

You can make your own massage oil by mixing 10 drops of essential oil in 2 tablespoons of carrier oil such as olive or grapeseed oil.

Make your point. For carpal tunnel syndrome, try this acupressure technique: Place the thumb of your right hand on the inside of your left wrist crease. (If your right wrist hurts more, work that side first.) Place your right index finger on the back of your left wrist, opposite your right thumb. Probe for the most sensitive area, then apply firm pressure to both sides of your wrist, alternating 5 seconds on and 5 seconds off. At the same time, gently move your left hand from side to side.

To increase the pain-reducing effect, exhale or blow through your mouth when you apply pressure. Continue on-and-off applications for 1 minute. Repeat on your right wrist if necessary.

Limber those digits. To stretch the muscles and tendons in your fingers, gently press your fingertips against the edge of a desk or table, bending at the base of your fingers and keeping your wrists straight. Once you feel the stretch, hold that position until you notice a change in sensation. Vary the exercise by doing it with your fingers spread apart.

Pose against pain. A yoga posture called the downward-facing dog creates the best skeletal alignment between the forearm and arm as well as between the shoulder and upper arm. Stand in front of a chair and put your palms flat on the front edge of the seat about shoulder-width apart. Spread your fingers so that your middle fingers are parallel and in line with your wrists. Move your feet backward until they're under your hips and your arms are straight. Bend your knees and point your tailbone toward the ceiling, creating a gentle arch in your lower back. Lower your head so that your ears are between your upper arms.

Keep your hands parallel as you slide them away from your body toward the back of the chair, straighten your knees, and balance your weight between your upper and lower body. You will feel a lengthening stretch extend from your shoulders to your wrists. Take a deep breath and hold for 15 to 30 seconds. Repeat 3 to 10 times a day. With practice, this pose will become easier and you can try turning your shoulders out and away from your neck, broadening your upper back as you stretch.

Sciatica

Sciatica gets on your nerves in more ways than one. When you have the condition, almost every move you make is painful—standing, sitting, even hoisting a half-gallon of milk.

Most cases of sciatica result from some irritation of the sciatic nerve, which originates in the spinal cord and branches throughout both legs.

What sorts of things irritate the sciatic nerve? Often, the gel-like contents of a spinal disk leak out and press on the nerve. Arthritis in the spine may pinch the nerve. Or chemicals produced by your body in response to a lower-back injury may inflame the nerve.

Sciatica pain can last for up to a month or so. Here's what you can do to help move it out.

Create some space. Sit on the forward part of a sturdy chair with your feet flat on the floor and your back straight. Slowly tilt your pelvis backward so that your lower back is slightly rounded; relax. Next, slowly tilt your pelvis forward so that your lower back arches; relax. Repeat four to eight times, then return to the starting position. Tilt your pelvis toward your left knee so that your weight shifts to the forward part of your left buttock; relax. Do the same toward your right knee; relax. Repeat four to eight times.

Hit the shower. If your sciatica is caused by a muscle strain, a muscle spasm, or another lower-back injury, try stretching in the shower. Begin by standing with your back to the spray and letting warm water run over your body for 5 to 10 minutes. Gently lean forward from your waist to the point just before pain sets in. (Hold on to a grab bar or another sturdy structure so that you don't fall.) Stay in this position for several seconds before slowly straightening up. Stand upright for a few seconds, then repeat. Finally, do the same movement to each side.

Stretch. Avoid sitting for long periods. Stretching stimulates circulation and reduces inflammation. Stretch every 30 minutes.

Get on your feet. Walking for 3 to 5 minutes of every hour makes sciatica heal faster.

Limit heat. Refrain from using a heating pad or soaking in a hot bath for longer than 30 minutes. Too much heat can increase swelling and aggravate pain. Instead, opt for a cold pack wrapped in a towel every few hours for 10 to 15 minutes.

Shoulder Pain

Folks often get shoulder pain from taking on tasks that tax their shoulder muscles. When these muscles aren't used much, they stiffen and lose their flexibility. Then, when they're put to work—say, cleaning out kitchen cupboards or going for a swim—they balk big-time.

Sometimes shoulder muscles become pinched between the bones and ligaments in your back, a painful condition called impingement. Then there's adhesive capsulitis, in which the shoulder stiffens so much that it can't move.

Here's what you can do to get your shoulder back in the swing of things.

Stop what you're doing. At the first sign of shoulder pain, stop whatever you're doing. To ignore means you're asking for more.

Ice it. Wrap ice or an ice pack in a towel and apply it to your sore shoulder for no more than 20 minutes of each hour. The cold reduces inflammation.

Preserve your flexibility. Once your acute pain subsides, try this exercise sequence to restore your shoulder's range of motion. Begin with your arm hanging at your side. Raise it in front of you until it's over your head (or until you feel pain), then lower it. Repeat 10 times. Raise your arm out to the side, then lower it. Repeat 10 times. Tuck your upper arm against your body and bend your elbow so that your forearm is in front of you. Move your forearm toward your stomach, then return to the starting position. Repeat 10 times. Finally, rotate your forearm to the outside, then return to the starting position. Repeat 10 times. Practice the entire sequence once or twice each day, as long as you don't feel pain.

Tendinitis and Bursitis

With names like tennis elbow, housemaid's knees, and weaver's bottom, it sounds more like a Martha Stewart gardenwear collection than like a bunch of bruised joints. Both tendinitis and bursitis are painful inflammations in and around the elbow, knee, hip, or any other joint that is put through repeated pressure and activity.

While both conditions are painful enough to sideline you, they will get better on their own. If you don't improve after 3 to 4 days, see your doctor. If you want a speedier recovery, try the following natural remedies.

Stop it. Some women are so stubborn that they'll just try to keep right on going through the pain. Don't. It'll only prolong the agony.

Put the pain on ice. Wrap ice or an ice pack in a towel and apply it to the affected area for up to 20 minutes. Repeat three or four times a day.

Give yourself a raise. Elevating the affected area above heart level alleviates swelling. So if your ankle hurts, slide a pillow or two underneath it, then lie down.

Promote healing with herbs. Ginger has potent anti-inflammatory properties. To make a tea from the dried herb, mix about ½ teaspoon ginger with 1 cup boiled water, then steep for 20 minutes.

Keep moving. Pampering the affected area too much can leave it stiff and prone to reinjury if it's not up to the task that you set for it. So once the initial pain subsides, continuously do gentle exercises to keep the area flexible.

Toothache

Any number of things can make a tooth hurt. But most often, the culprit is tooth decay.

A toothache should never be ignored. If you get one, call your dentist right away. The following remedies can keep you comfortable until you get proper medical attention.

Swoosh and spit. If the area around a tooth begins to swell, rinse your mouth with warm water. The water just might flush out debris that's irritating your gums.

Try some cloves. Put a drop of clove oil on your aching tooth. Clove oil acts as a local anesthetic and antiseptic. You'll find clove oil in health food stores.

Soothe with spices. Mix ground ginger or ground red pepper (or both) in enough water to make a gooey paste. Dip a cotton ball in the paste, squeeze out any excess, and then apply the cotton directly to the sore tooth. The heat generated by this remedy acts as a counterirritant to the deeper pain. Don't let the paste touch your gums, though, because it can be very irritating to sensitive tissue.

If this mini-compress feels too hot, rinse your mouth and discontinue use.

Make a move. Twenty-five minutes of aerobic activity can trigger the release of endorphins, feel-good brain chemicals that can temporarily help subdue the pain.

Fast First-Aid

Accidents happen. And for many of us, they happen in the kitchen.

Charlotte S. Yeh, M.D., rates the kitchen as one of the most hazardous rooms in the home. "Cooking, washing dishes, and even taking out the trash can lead to burns, cuts, and similar minor injuries," says Dr. Yeh, an emergency physician at the New England Medical Center in Boston. Another risky area is the bathroom. "Older women, in particular, are prone to falls in the bathroom that sometimes result in sprains," she notes.

Of course, minor medical emergencies—from cuts and scrapes to burns and bruises—occur not only at home but also on the job, on the road, and on playing fields. The best way to be prepared to handle them is to have a well-stocked first-aid kit at home and in your car. Dr. Yeh suggests that you include the following items.

- Adhesive bandages
- Antibiotic cream and/or ointment
- Chemical cold packs

- Disposable gloves
- Elastic bandages
- Gauze and adhesive tape
- List of emergency phone numbers
- Scissors with rounded tips (to cut bandages to fit)
- Triangular bandage (to make a sling)
- Tweezers

To complete your kit, add a bottle of ipecac syrup (an antidote for poisoning), a small bottle of tea tree essential oil (a natural antiseptic), a few 500-milligram capsules of ginger (to relieve motion sickness or nausea), and a bottle of homeopathic Arnica 30C (for bumps, bruises, and muscle strains), recommends Connie Catellani, M.D., medical director at the Miro Center for Integrative Medicine in Evanston, Illinois. With these items handy, you will be ready to handle any minor emergency fast, if you know what to do. So read on to learn how to become an amateur at-home first-aid administrator.

Bee Stings

Bee stings aren't always just a casual mishap of summer. Some people can have life-threatening allergic reactions to bee stings. If you develop hives that start to multiply on your body and experience any trouble breathing, intense anxiety, allover itching or swelling, dizziness, weakness, or sweating, get to the emergency room at once. It could mean that you are going through a severe and sometimes fatal hypersensitivity reaction known as anaphylactic shock and need a shot of adrenaline immediately. (Some people who know they are allergic carry bee sting kits with them.) For run-of-the-mill stings, here's what to do.

FOLK REMEDY: DOES IT WORK?

Mud on a Bee Sting

Why mud works on bee stings isn't completely understood. It probably has something to do with its drying effect, according to Connie Catellani, M.D., medical director at the Miro Center for Integrative Medicine in Evanston, Illinois. As the mud dries, it helps to cool the sting site, which brings pain relief. It may also draw out a stinger that has been left behind.

The next time you are stung by a bee, remove the stinger immediately, if possible. Then mix some dirt in the palm of your hand with clean water until you have mud. (Soil that has a lot of clay in it works best.) The mud should be thick enough to coat the affected area but not so thick that you can't feel it drying. Put the mud on the sting and let it dry, states Dr. Catellani. Leave it in place until it starts to crumble off, usually in 1 to 2 hours. One application is all that's necessary.

Recommendation: Worth a Try

Do some home surgery. If you are stung by a honeybee, remove the stinger—the sooner the better. Using a credit card, a dull knife, or the back of your thumbnail, scrape your skin beneath the stinger until it comes out. Avoid squeezing around the fuzzy part of the stinger. That's the venom sac, and if you break it, you will release even more venom.

Cover with a cool compress. Soak a washcloth in cool water. Then lay it on the site of the sting to ease soreness and itching.

Put it on ice. To relieve swelling and pain, hold an ice cube on the sting for a few minutes, remove it for a few minutes, then repeat. Continue for no longer than 10 minutes. (You don't want to harm your skin.)

Apply a healing paste. Mix a paste of baking soda and water, then apply it to the site of the sting to neutralize acidity.

Raise the area. If the sting becomes so swollen that it aches, elevate the affected body part. Gravity will draw fluid from the area, reducing the swelling and the associated soreness.

Burns

Dripping grease, hot handles, simmering liquid, even the waffle iron all can create a red, throbbing, painful burn that can last for hours.

These are known as first-degree burns and can be treated easily at home, according to Jonith Breadon, M.D., a dermatologist and codirector of dermatological surgery at the dermatology residency program at Cook County Hospital in Chicago. If a burn is blistered, you could have a second- or even third-degree burn. Get medical attention immediately.

To stop the burn of a minor mishap, do this.

Soak it—pronto! Hold the burned area under cool running water for at least 15 minutes. If you aren't close to a faucet, then use whatever you have handy to cool the burn—even a cold can of soda wrapped in a clean towel. Rinse the area with cool water as soon as you are able.

Cleanse and protect. Gently wash the affected area twice each day, using either mild soap or hydrogen peroxide. Don't use hydrogen peroxide for more than 3 days, however—prolonged use can actually impair wound healing. Apply an over-the-counter antibacterial ointment, then cover the area with an adhesive strip (for small burns) or a gauze dressing (for large burns).

FOLK REMEDY: DOES IT WORK?

Butter for a Burn

"Slathering a burn with butter does not reduce the pain or stop the burning," says Mary Ruth Buchness, M.D., chief of dermatology at St. Vincent's Hospital and Medical Center in New York City.

In fact, putting butter on a burn could lead to infection, warns Dr. Buchness. Because burned skin has lost its protective top layer, it is vulnerable to infection-causing bacteria. And food products—butter included—are often teeming with bacteria.

Recommendation: Forget It

Go for aloe. If you have an aloe vera plant, break off a leaf and rub the gel from inside the leaf on your burn. Or use aloe vera cream, available in drugstores and health food stores.

Moisturize the site. Once the burn has healed, regularly apply a thin layer of moisturizer to reduce itching and cracking and promote healing. Choose a fragrance-free lotion.

Increase your C intake. Vitamin C rebuilds collagen, the skin's connective tissue, and speeds healing.

Cuts and Scrapes

When you have a break in your skin, its natural repair system leaps into action, quite literally. Researchers have microscopically witnessed cells moving about to fill in wounds. You can help the process along by taking steps to prevent infection and promote healing. Here's how.

Wash away debris. To prevent infection, hold a cut or scrape under running water until it is thoroughly cleaned.

Don't use hydrogen peroxide for this purpose—it kills healthy skin cells that promote healing.

Coat with a natural ointment. Apply calendula ointment directly to the wound. Calendula has antiseptic properties. You can buy the ointment in health food stores.

Cover up. Covering the wound with an adhesive bandage keeps it clean and dry and speeds healing. Change the bandage twice a day.

Slip into your second skin. As an alternative to a bandage, try an over-the-counter product called colloidal dressing. This porous, gelatin-like material sticks to your skin, creating a breathable membrane over the wound. Plus, it contains an antimicrobial medication, which fights infection. Experts say that these dressings can cut healing time in half.

Make a soothing spray. Mix 15 drops of lavender essential oil with 2 tablespoons of aloe vera juice (available in health food stores). Pour the solution into a spray bottle and refrigerate. Spray on the cut or scrape as often as necessary to ease pain while you heal.

Frostbite

Most people think of frostbite as a cold-weather hazard. But the air doesn't have to be all that cold for frostbite to occur. High winds can reduce temperatures to dangerously low levels, what we know as the windchill factor. So even if the thermometer says 20°F, a 40-mile-per-hour wind can create a windchill index of –20°F conditions. And frostbite can happen at a temperature of just 10°F.

Your hands, feet, ears, nose, and other extremities are the first to feel the chill. Once your skin freezes, small, icy crystals form and destroy the skin cells. This causes your blood to clot, cutting off circulation to the area. Your flesh hardens, your skin becomes waxy and white, and you lose all feeling in the affected area.

If you suspect that you have frostbite, treat it immediately by following these steps. And see your doctor as soon as possible—you can't tell how serious the damage is just by looking at your skin.

Seek shelter. If you notice your skin turning waxy white, get inside before frostbite develops in other areas. If you can't head indoors and you are with someone, cozy up to keep your extremities warm. Sharing body heat can help prevent frostnip (when your skin is numb and cold but not frozen) from developing into frostbite.

Loosen up. As your skin thaws, it will swell. So once you are inside, remove all constrictive clothing and jewelry.

Leave the area alone. Rubbing frostbitten skin does more damage. Don't even touch it.

Don't refreeze it. Frostbite does its harm when your skin thaws, then refreezes. So don't thaw out your skin unless you know you are staying inside.

Stay away from fire. Your frozen nerve endings won't be able to warn you if you start to burn your skin, so don't try to warm yourself over a flame.

Get into warm water. Once you are certain that you won't refreeze the affected area, gradually immerse it in a tub or saucepan of warm (102° to 105°F) water. Circulate the water to help keep it in contact with your frozen body part and replenish the warmth continually. Warming frostbitten fingers and toes can be painful.

Once you have seen your doctor and are on the road to recovery, try these steps to aid healing.

- Rub fresh gel from an aloe vera plant on the frostbitten area. Aloe works against thromboxanes, substances that constrict blood vessels. When the vessels relax, the frostbitten area heals faster.

- Bandage fresh sliced beets onto the frostbitten area to ease pain and tenderness. Leave the beets on until they are dry. Repeat as necessary.

Insect Bites

Most insect bites are uncomfortable nuisances but not health hazards. To relieve the redness, swelling, and itching, try these natural remedies.

Come clean. Thoroughly wash a bite with soap and water to remove germs and allergy-provoking substances.

Make it ice-cold. For swelling and itching, rub an ice cube over the welt for a few minutes at a time. Repeat throughout the day as necessary. (Avoid leaving the ice in one area for more than a few minutes. It can damage your skin.)

Take a soak. To minimize itching, add colloidal oatmeal to a tub of lukewarm water, then climb in and soak. You can buy colloidal oatmeal in drugstores.

Make your own repellent. Add the following essential oils to ¼ cup of vegetable oil: five drops of eucalyptus, two drops of rosemary, four drops of lavender, two drops of juniper, eight drops of cedar, one drop of peppermint, one drop of clove, and one drop of cinnamon. Pour into a glass spray bottle, mix thoroughly, and apply liberally to discourage bugs from making a meal out of you. Look for essential oils in health food stores.

Motion Sickness

Motion sickness occurs when your brain receives conflicting messages about the movement affecting your body. For example, if you are in the cabin of a boat and you can't see the choppy waves outside, everything looks still. But your inner ears and your legs sense the boat's movement. When your brain receives these conflicting messages, you feel sick.

Probably the most annoying symptom of motion sickness is the stomach distress—the queasiness, nausea, and

Get the Tick Off—Carefully

A tick's bite is generally painless, and a tick sticks around as long as it can, burrowing its head into your skin, where it quietly feasts on your blood. Some ticks carry Lyme disease and Rocky Mountain spotted fever.

"Somewhere between 48 and 72 hours after a tick attaches itself to your skin, the various disease-causing bacteria it may carry will begin to pass into your body. So it is important to check for ticks regularly and remove them promptly," explains Ada Huang, M.D., deputy commissioner for disease control at the Westchester County Health Department in New Rochelle, New York.

Avoid using folk remedies rumored to coax ticks out or kill them, says Dr. Huang. Applying lotions or ointments might spread the bacteria. Instead, keep the tick intact; if it ruptures, the bacteria it carries could spread. Dr. Huang suggests using extra-fine-tip tweezers to grasp the tick as close as possible to your skin. Apply steady, firm pressure and pull the tick away from the skin. Do not squeeze or twist the tick.

After the tick is out, wash the bite with soap and water, disinfect the area with rubbing alcohol, and apply a topical first-aid antibiotic ointment. See a physician if any unusual symptoms appear. For Lyme disease, regularly examine the area for the next 30 days. If a rash appears or if you develop flulike symptoms (fever or muscle aches without a runny nose and sore throat), see a physician.

vomiting. Other symptoms include dizziness, faintness, fatigue, sweating, difficulty breathing, and even blackouts.

The quickest cure for motion sickness is to plant your feet on terra firma. Of course, that's not always possible, so here are remedies that can quiet your stomach in a jiffy.

Keep your eyes open. When you focus on something outside of the boat or vehicle and watch where you are going, the cues from your eyes more closely match the cues from your inner ears. This reduces your likelihood of getting sick.

Control your breathing. When you are in a situation that may bring on motion sickness, alter your breathing by inhaling for 2 seconds and exhaling for 2 seconds. This technique switches off your body's stress response, so you are less likely to become sick.

Get to the point. Press down on the middle of the crease of your wrist on the inside, just below your palm, with your thumb. Press fairly hard for about 10 minutes. This acupressure technique inhibits nausea and dizziness.

Break out the band. You can duplicate the effects of the acupressure technique described above with a modern wristband called a Sea-Band. It works by pressing a plastic stud into the middle of the underside of each wrist.

Snap up ginger. Ginger settles the stomach, so it can help relieve motion sickness. Take one or two capsules of powdered ginger (sold in health food stores) three times a day while you are traveling.

Eat a little before leaving. Consuming a light meal within 2 to 3 hours of traveling can keep motion sickness at bay.

Choose wisely. Where you sit in a moving vehicle can determine whether or not you get sick. Choose locations with a view of the horizon and the least motion, such as the front seat of a car, the center deck of a boat, and a window seat near the wing on an airplane.

Nosebleed

For such a small body part, the nose can spill a lot of blood. That's because the blood vessels that serve your nose are very close to the surface, so they rupture with the slightest provocation.

You can almost always stop a nosebleed on your own. Here's how.

Squeeze it dry. Using your thumb and forefinger, squeeze your nostrils shut for 5 minutes while tilting your head forward. If bleeding resumes, squeeze your nostrils shut, this time for 15 minutes. (If you can't stop the bleeding after 15 minutes, get to a doctor.)

Get a cold nose. If you have been hit in the nose, wrap a bag of ice cubes in a towel, then lie down on your side and hold the ice pack to your nose.

Get cottonmouth. Roll a piece of tissue or a cotton ball and place it in your mouth, right under your nose, between your upper lip and gums. Leave it there for 5 to 10 minutes. The cotton applies pressure to the blood vessels that send blood to your nose.

Forget stuffing. Putting a wad of cotton in a bloody nose only aggravates the bleeding. The cotton attaches to the scab inside your nose. When you remove the cotton, you remove the scab, and you start to bleed again.

Don't be a blowhard. Once your nose stops bleeding, refrain from blowing your nose.

Eat your C rations. Vitamin C supports the manufacture of collagen and mucus, substances that maintain the moist, protective lining inside your nose. If you are prone to nosebleeds, you should be sure to get at least 60 milligrams of vitamin C a day (the Daily Value), which can be obtained from C-rich foods and supplements.

Poison Ivy

It is the scourge of hikers, gardeners, and the country gentry.

If you have been exposed to poison ivy (or oak or sumac), the following tips can minimize your chances of experiencing a reaction and provide relief if you do get a rash.

Rinse off with rubbing alcohol. Stay outdoors and liberally splash all exposed areas of your body with rubbing alcohol. (Be careful to keep it away from your eyes.) Then wash off the alcohol with a garden hose. But act fast—you may have only a few minutes before the oil seeps into your skin.

Disrobe in the laundry room. As soon as you can, remove all of your clothing and thoroughly wash it in hot, soapy water. Wash your shoes, too—or at least rinse them off.

Create a milk compress. Soak a washcloth or a piece of gauze in cold milk, then hold it against your skin.

Dab on witch hazel. Soak a cotton ball in witch hazel, then apply the clear liquid to the affected area of your skin.

Discover a jewel. The herb jewelweed reduces the inflammation associated with poison ivy rash just as well as cortisone creams do. You can buy jewelweed cream in health food stores.

Sprains

Many doctors say that sprains can be more complicated than broken bones. Most simple, garden-variety breaks are easy to fix. You just push them back in place (sometimes surgically) until they mend together. Sprains can be a different matter altogether.

A sprain requires 2 to 8 weeks to heal completely, depending on how bad it is. You can assist the process by pampering the injured joint and following these tips.

Is It Broken?

You slip and fall on the ice and hurt your leg. Or you tumble down the stairs and land solidly on your arm. The pain is excruciating. Your first thoughts: Is it broken? I have to get to a hospital or emergency center.

But wait. If you even suspect a break, the first caveat is "Don't move," says Constance Nichols, M.D., emergency physician at the University of Massachusetts Medical Center in Worcester. Assess the damage first.

Bruising and swelling aren't always the best indicators of whether or not a bone is broken. A bad sprain can be very swollen, while a fracture may be only slightly swollen—at least at first. "Even doctors can't always tell a sprain from a break," says Dr. Nichols.

If the injury seems less severe, put ice on it and keep the limb elevated. If you don't get some relief within 12 to 24 hours, see your doctor.

A limb that may be broken needs to be kept still to prevent further injury.

To get to the hospital under your own steam, you need to splint the injury to prevent further damage. You can make a homemade splint using anything that's straight and stiff, such as a closed umbrella, a golf club, short lengths of wood, cardboard, a thick magazine, several thicknesses of newspaper, or a pillow tied with a belt or rope. Be sure to loosen the splint if swelling increases or if the area beyond the splint becomes pale or numb or throbs.

Get off it. Putting weight on a sprained ligament can turn a partial tear into a full one. So immediately get the injured joint up and out of harm's way.

Just add ice. Wrap ice in a cloth and apply it to the sprain for 20 minutes. Reapply the ice pack every few

Use a pillow splint to stabilize an ankle, wrist, or hand. Position the limb in a relaxed pose on top of a pillow and then wrap the pillow around it. Secure the splint with several strips of cloth or anything else you can tie around it to hold it in place, and then elevate.

Use a thick magazine to splint the upper arm. Roll the magazine around the arm and secure it with strips of cloth or anything else you can tie around it to hold it in place. To support the weight of the arm, make a sling by tying the ends of a long strip of cloth around your neck. The bottom of the loop should hang at about waist level so you can easily slip the forearm through it and keep the elbow at about a 90-degree angle. For further support, splint the arm to your chest with a strip of cloth.

Use a heavy cardboard splint for a broken forearm. It keeps the arm from rotating. Fold the cardboard in thirds so that it "sandwiches" the arm, with cardboard coming up both sides. Be sure the cardboard is long enough to extend from the palm past the elbow. Place the cardboard around the injured arm, with the thumb pointing up, and secure it with strips of cloth or anything else you can tie around it to hold it in place. Once the splint is on, follow the directions above for making a sling and chest splint to reduce further movement.

hours until the pain and swelling subside. (Avoid putting ice directly on your skin. It can cause frostbite.)

Wrap it up. Use an elastic bandage to compress the area around the sprained joint. This reduces swelling.

Elevate. Raise the injured joint above heart level to minimize pain and swelling.

Aid with arnica. Apply arnica cream to the sprained area as soon as possible after the injury to reduce pain, swelling, and bruising. Repeat three or four times a day for 5 days. This herbal cream is available in most health food stores.

Note: Don't use arnica on broken skin or open wounds. And don't get it in your eyes.

Part Two

Look Your Best

Win at Weight Loss

The funny thing about dieting is that it's a pretty easy concept to grasp: Take in fewer calories than you put out, and you lose weight. Eat more than you burn, and you gain. In practice, though, it's an entirely different story.

One reason is that food is irresistible. For reasons too many and too complicated to go into here, people find comfort in eating and, quite often, in eating too much of the wrong thing at the wrong time.

Food is central to the good side of life. It's good food and drink (and, of course, good company) that bring festivity to celebrations, parties, family gatherings, and holidays. So it's not so easy to take in less than you use up. Present-day lifestyles aren't helping any, either.

"We are actually exercising less," says Susan Zelitch Yanovski, M.D., director of the obesity and eating disorders program in the division of digestive diseases and nutrition at the National Institute of Diabetes and Digestive and Kidney Diseases. "We sit at our jobs all day. We drive everywhere. We're eating as though we're doing a lot of physical activity, but we're not expending that kind of energy."

In addition, our bodies' calorie-burning mechanisms—our metabolisms—are slowing as we age. After age 30, we burn 2 to 4 percent fewer calories every 10 years. Compound that with less exercise and more reasons to eat, and the scale goes up and up.

Unfortunately, there's no magic pill to melt away fat. But there is a successful formula: Healthy eating + exercise + motivation = success. "The weight comes off more gradually—about 1 to 2 pounds per week," says Dr. Yanovski. "Do it slow and easy, and it may be more likely to stay off."

It really doesn't have to be very hard. Here are tips from the country's top weight-loss experts on how to eat and exercise for weight loss and where to get the motivation to follow through.

Low-Fat Living

Gram for gram, dietary fat supplies more calories than carbohydrates—9 calories per gram of fat versus 4 calories per gram of carbohydrate. And fat calories are more easily stored by the body than carbohydrate calories.

The rule of thumb is that you should limit your daily fat intake to 25 percent of calories. That not only makes good weight-loss sense but also is good for your overall health. For a person who consumes 1,500 calories a day, for example, no more than 375 calories should come from fat. (That's about 41 grams of fat.)

To get an idea of how much fat and how many calories you consume daily, take one typical day and jot down everything you eat. Then count up the calories and fat, using a dependable fat-and-calorie counter. Check labels on the things you're eating, too; you'll find all the numbers you need on the packages.

Based on your findings, change your eating habits according to these tips. You'll cut back on fat automatically.

Become a part-time vegetarian. Giving up animal foods is the single easiest way to cut fat and calories. And you don't even have to go whole hog, so to speak. Just eating one or two meatless meals per week will help.

Give meat a supporting role. When you do include meat in your meals, treat it as a side dish rather than as the main course. Think of your dinner plate as having three compartments, like one of those divided paper plates. Put the meat in one of the smaller compartments. Fill the big one with vegetables. Put grains in the remaining compartment, allowing them to spill over into the veggies. Redesigning your plate in this way automatically slashes fat grams and calories to healthy levels.

Halve the fat in home cooking. You can eliminate as much as half of the fat from a recipe without altering its taste. Substitute kidney beans for half of the meat in chili. Replace half of the cheese in lasagna with spinach. Trade in sour cream for yogurt in casseroles, sauces, and dips. Use applesauce instead of some or all of the oil or margarine in cakes, muffins, and breads. Experiment with quantities until you're satisfied with the taste and texture.

Add a bit of butter. Using just 1 teaspoon of butter wisely can satisfy your tastebuds. For instance, add fresh chopped herbs to 1 teaspoon of melted butter to create a richly flavored topping for broiled fish.

Keep healthy foods handy. If you work in an office, stock your desk with low-fat foods such as single-serving cans of tuna and dehydrated soups. Then, on days when you don't have time to pack your lunch, you have a fast and healthful meal right at your fingertips. You won't be as tempted to head for the nearest vending machine or fast-food outlet for a bite to eat.

Use a fork, not your fingers. How many cookies and potato chips can you eat with a fork? Except for raw fruits and vegetables, avoid finger foods. They're usually loaded with fat—and because they pop into your mouth so easily, you'll likely eat more than you should.

Find new favorites. Don't eat foods that you don't like, even if they're low-fat and nutritious. Forcing yourself to eat something that you hate may turn you off to healthy eating.

Eating Out

Eating out used to be a luxury. These days, it's practically a necessity, making it the number-one saboteur of all your best intentions. That's because you're at the mercy of a chef, possibly one with a penchant for a little extra butter or cream or other "taste enhancers."

Some establishments identify certain menu items as low-fat or low-calorie. And they're now required to back up such nutrition claims, thanks to the FDA's truth-in-menu regulations. But a chef won't always stick with the recipe that was used to evaluate fat-and-calorie content. So you still don't know what you're getting.

Even nutrition experts have a hard time estimating the fat-and-calorie content of restaurant fare. In one study, a group that included dietitians underestimated the fat in five restaurant meals by an average of 49 percent.

Consider the following your own truth-in-ordering regulations.

First, have a drink. Of water, that is. A large glass of ice-cold water will help start filling you up, so you'll be less likely to overeat. Sip while you peruse the menu, and drink generously throughout the meal.

Make certain words off-limits. In general, avoid any dish described in the menu as breaded, scalloped, crispy, fried, au gratin, or creamy. These foods are almost certain to be high in fat or calories.

Make a special request. Tell your server exactly how you want your food prepared—for example, without oil or butter. The vast majority of restaurants say they will change the way they prepare a dish at a customer's request.

Say, "On the side, please." Always ask that a sauce or salad dressing be served on the side. That way, you control how much you eat. Dip your fork into the sauce or dressing, then stab a morsel of meat or several leaves of lettuce. You get all of the flavor but not as much fat.

Turn down the freebies. Many restaurants serve tortilla chips, crispy noodles, or other munchies to tide over customers until their meals arrive. Just set them aside. Or tell your server not to bring them in the first place. Bread is okay, as long as you resist the urge to slather it with butter.

Eat half as much. Restaurant portions are usually big enough to feed two people. Before you dig in to your entrée, set aside half of it to take home, and ask the server to put it in a doggie bag. If you want an appetizer or dessert, share it with your dining companion.

Bingeing

Some folks become so fat conscious that they forget the positive and pleasurable aspects of eating. They eat salads for lunch and plain broiled fish for dinner day after day. This monotony can lead to mad fat cravings, which can turn into a full-blown binge.

A binge also can be emotionally driven. Spats at home or a bad day at work can turn into romancing with food. It has long been known that food is solace for negative feelings—usually anger, anxiety, or depression.

It wouldn't be so bad if it happened occasionally and then you got right back to your good intentions. But bingeing makes you feel even worse about yourself and sets up a vicious cycle. For some, binges can last for days. Here are some ways to binge-proof your body and mind.

Eat! Starving yourself is a sure route to bingeing. Instead, start each day by filling your empty stomach with a breakfast of satiating protein, appetite-curbing fiber, and energy-boosting carbohydrates.

Eat a little, a lot. Instead of eating three squares a day, consider dividing your typical meals into mini-meals every couple of hours. This will keep you from starving yourself between meals, and, even though it seems contrary to logic, you'll end up eating less.

Pay attention to what you're eating. When you inhale a bagel or a sandwich in your car or at your desk, you don't really enjoy the food. So, later, you're more likely to crave the flavor experience that you missed in the first place. Instead, take time to focus on what you're eating. Savor every bite.

Plan indulgences. Buy one serving of a favorite "forbidden" food—one that's intensely flavored and long lasting, such as a half-ounce of rich gourmet chocolate. Let the chocolate melt on your tongue and give it a lot of mouth play. By allowing yourself to enjoy a little of the food, you can thwart an all-out binge.

See yourself rejecting food. Visualize a situation that makes you vulnerable to bingeing. For example, imagine that you're going to be home alone with half a cheesecake left over from a recent party. See and smell the cheesecake. Let the craving develop. Then see yourself destroying the cheesecake or putting it in the freezer, out of sight. Practice this visualization technique two or three times a day to control bingeing.

Use your "D" fences. If you feel a binge coming on, use the five Ds to try to ride it out.

1. Determine what's going on. Ask yourself, "Why is my desire to eat so high right now? Am I sad, angry, lonely, in conflict?"
2. Delay your response by figuring out what is tempting you. Do you have trouble resisting lures like a party's festive buffet table or the smell of fresh baked goods?
3. Distract yourself for 10 minutes.
4. Distance yourself from the temptation. Either remove yourself or have someone remove the temptation from you.
5. Decide what positive steps you can take right now and in the future to strengthen your willpower.

Match your food to your mood. If you give in to the urge to binge, choose a low-fat food that matches how you're feeling. If you're angry, for example, reach for something crunchy, such as pretzels or raw veggies. If you're feeling blue, go for smooth, creamy yogurt or pudding.

Savor something spicy. Hard as you may try, you just can't binge on chile peppers or hot-pepper sauce. Plus, spicy foods fill you up faster than bland or sweet foods.

Freeze the moment. You've given in to a binge, and you're about to feel like a failure. Don't. Stop and think about why you're using food inappropriately. If you've polished off half a bag of buttered popcorn, acknowledge your stuffed feeling. Then get up and toss out the rest. By tuning in to your bingeing and freezing the moment, you can stop the binge. And even if you don't stop eating, you have a chance to control how much you eat the next time.

Go easy on yourself. An evening of out-of-control eating doesn't mean that you should toss out your weight-loss goals. It just means that you've gotten sidetracked. Self-forgiveness is the first step in learning and moving on.

Face your slipup squarely and ask yourself what you've learned from it. Success or failure is not about how badly you fall down but about how well you pick yourself up and recover.

Beating the Hungries

You've eaten dinner, and you feel as stuffed as the flounder that was on your plate. You swear you couldn't eat another bite. Then the dessert cart rolls up, and before you know it, you're ordering death-by-chocolate torte.

What's going on is that you're confusing hunger, the gnawing urge to eat that you feel after a several-hour fast, with appetite, the desire to eat whether you're hungry or not. And it's appetite, not hunger, that gets you into trouble.

Appetite is a response to external cues, and in some people, it overreacts. It may tell you to eat because the clock says you should or because you're at the movies or because your coworker just showed up with a box of doughnuts.

Recognizing the difference between hunger and appetite is important to your weight-loss success. If you eat only when you're hungry and stop when you're really full, excess grams of fat and calories shouldn't be an issue. Granted, appetite is a mighty strong force to reckon with. Here are some tips to get it under control.

Minimize your meals. This bears repeating. Divide your meals into five or six smaller meals. Without long absences of food, your appetite will be more content.

Chew food thoroughly. It takes about 20 minutes for the food you eat to enter your bloodstream as glucose (blood sugar) and turn off hunger. So slowly chew each morsel of food 10 to 15 times before swallowing. This allows you to truly savor your food and also helps with its digestion. Besides, the effort you put into chewing every bite thoroughly will make you less inclined to overeat.

Munch to Mozart. Listening to music during a meal helps you to focus on what you're eating, and the rhythm helps you slow down. Choose slow, calming tunes; a fast beat may make you eat faster and "forget" what you've eaten.

No TV dinners. Research shows that people who watch television while eating tend to eat significantly more than people who don't. That's because we're more intent on what we're watching than on what we're eating. And that doesn't suit a demanding appetite.

Go easy on the fat. Eating a high-fat meal may leave you craving even more fat, research suggests. A study found that laboratory animals that were fed meals of more than 40 percent fat continued to produce high levels of a neurochemical that induces fat cravings.

Chat more, eat less. Talking more and eating less is one expert's advice to prevent overindulging at mealtime. The conversation may pull your attention away from the food and add some time between each mouthful.

Help for Trouble Zones

You can diet all you want, but only exercise is going to trim the fleshy thighs, bigger bottom, and jelly belly you have acquired over the years.

Mother Nature once again can take the rap for bestowing women with these trouble zones. An enzyme called lipoprotein lipase actually directs fat to your hips, buttocks, and thighs for your body to use during pregnancy. Aging augments the problem. As you get older, your body produces less collagen and elastin, the connective tissues that enable skin to stretch and contract. Without these substances, your skin starts to sag, taking on a flabby appearance.

The good news is that you can sculpt your body's trouble zones. In addition to maintaining a healthful diet, though, you must exercise steadily and aerobically as well as do some resistance training. Here are the basics to get you started.

Why Cellulite Is a Women's Problem

Cellulite is the dimply fat that congregates on many women's thighs, buttocks, or hips. Men don't get it because they have thicker, more resilient skin than women. The fibers that anchor skin to muscle are configured differently in men than in women. In men, the fibers crisscross to form a tight net that holds fat firmly in place. In women, the fibers run in only one direction. The combination of sagging skin and slack fibers allows fat to bulge outward, creating cellulite's trademark "cottage cheese" appearance.

Another reason men don't have a problem with cellulite is that they tend to carry their weight around their midriffs. Fat in this area is firmer and more dimple proof than fat on the lower body, where women tend to carry their weight.

To make cellulite less noticeable—or stop it from showing up in the first place—cut your calorie intake enough to produce a significant weight loss. That means cutting down on all calories, not just fat, and exercising regularly. Make sure that your workout includes 30 minutes of heart-pumping activity, like cycling, running, or brisk walking, at least 3 days a week, plus muscle-building strength training on the off days. As your fat stores shrink and your muscle tone improves, cellulite-prone areas will become tauter and smoother.

Put your heart in it. *Aerobic* describes any activity that increases your heart rate, works your heart and lungs, and burns fat. Vigorous walking, jogging, and bicycling qualify, as do dancing and gardening. Aim for at least 30 minutes of aerobic exercise three times a week.

Add some resistance. Resistance training tones and strengthens muscle mass, the infrastructure of your trouble zones. It also gives your metabolism a long-term boost by prompting you to build more muscle, which in turn burns more calories even when you're at rest. Experts suggest that you alternate your aerobic and resistance-training workouts. So if you walk Mondays, Wednesdays, and Fridays, do resistance training on Tuesdays and Thursdays.

Aim for the abs. Abdominal fat is more metabolically active than lower-body fat, so it's easier to lose. Ordinary walking can help, but try to put in some additional effort. Add 10 to 15 extra minutes to your regular walking routine. You can also try these two classic ab exercises that will help work your upper and lower abdominal muscles. To start, do one set of 8 to 15 repetitions three times a week. Gradually add more sets as you progress, and work up to five times a week.

For your upper abs, lie on your back with your knees bent, your feet flat on the floor, and your arms at your sides. Press your lower back into the floor so that there is no space between your back and the floor. Slowly raise your head and shoulders from the floor and reach forward with your arms, curling your trunk as much as possible until your fingertips touch your knees. Hold for 5 to 10 seconds and then return to the starting position. To keep your chin away from your chest while you're doing this exercise, imagine you are holding a small ball beneath your chin.

For your lower abs, lie on your back with your knees bent and your arms crossed over your chest. Keeping your lower back flat and your knees bent, raise your legs off the floor until your calves are almost parallel to the floor. Flex your feet and hold this position for 10 to 20 seconds. Be sure to breathe while holding this position. Slowly lower your legs and repeat.

Motivation

No amount of good intention can possibly matter if you don't have the motivation to make it through the long haul. Motivation is everything. No, it isn't always going to be easy, but there are tons of people out there who persevered and have been successful at losing. Here are a few tips from them on how they made it happen.

Go by feel, not by the scale. Do your rings feel looser? Do your pants feel less tight around the waist? Watching yourself melt back into a favorite outfit is a much bigger motivator than watching the scale. Scales, in fact, have been found to be downright discouraging.

Take it easy. Many people sabotage themselves by expecting too much, too fast. Try for 2 pounds a week, max.

Reward your efforts. Each time you meet a goal, no matter how small, treat yourself to something special. Pampering is always a nice reward. Get a manicure or massage.

Don't get in a rut. Don't do the same thing over and over. For every milestone you hit, change the way you achieved it. For example, buy a new low-fat cookbook to get some new recipes. Or walk in the community park instead of around your neighborhood. Or choose a new tape to listen to while you're pedaling your stationary bike.

Picture yourself thin. Visualize yourself losing weight. Imagine how you would feel and what your body would look like. This programs the subconscious mind to do what you want.

Recruit a weight-loss buddy. By pairing up with someone, you become accountable to that person. So you're much less likely to blow off a workout. Choose someone who's at a similar level of fitness so that you can keep up with each other and share the satisfaction of each other's progress.

Losing the Last 5 Pounds

Pound by pound, inch by inch, you became slimmer and fitter—until you got to the dreaded last 5 pounds. It has been weeks and weeks, and you're beginning to believe they're here to stay.

Don't give up. You just need an extra nudge. What has happened is that your eating and exercise habits have stayed the same, but you haven't. You're smaller now. Your body needs fewer calories to function. So the weight-loss program that took you from, say, 160 pounds to 130 may not be enough to get you to your final goal.

You have to shake things up a little. You have to burn more calories. Don't worry; it's not as hard as it sounds. Here's what to do.

Recheck your portion size. As you've been slimming down, it's likely that you've goosed up your eating just a tad, which didn't matter until now. Spend a few weeks eating prepackaged low-fat meals. The food label will tell you exactly what you're getting.

Limit your snacks. The snacks you've been enjoying may have gotten you to the weight you are now, but they could be stopping you from moving on. So forgo the low-fat cookies and crackers. Instead, get acquainted with oranges, carrots, and air-popped popcorn.

Add some rev to your metabolism. Anything over 30 minutes is fat-burning time, so add just an extra 10 to 15 minutes to your workout.

Try something new. You're not the only one who gets bored riding a stationary bike. Your muscles do too. If you always work the same muscles in the same way, they become very efficient and don't burn as many calories as when you first started an activity. Work your muscles in new ways by cross-training. If you've been walking, try swimming. If you've been running, try cycling. No one activity should ever become too easy.

Change your routine. Find little ways to increase your physical activity throughout the day. If you walk to work, for example, tack an extra block onto your route. Take the stairs instead of the elevator. And when you go to the supermarket or mall, park your car at the far end of the parking lot.

Ageless Skin

By the time tiny creases and crinkles on your skin become visible, a lot of irreversible changes have already occurred. In fact, these changes began years earlier, in your late twenties and early thirties. And they will continue as you get older and your skin gets drier, less resilient, and more fragile.

It's called aging. You can't stop it, but you can slow it down.

Of all the things that influence the health and appearance of your skin, none is as destructive as the sun, according to Gloria Graham, M.D., a dermatologist in Morehead City, North Carolina. By one estimate, at least 80 percent of all visible skin aging results from a lifetime of repeated sun exposure.

Ageless Ideas

"To get some idea of the effects of sun exposure, take a look at the skin on your breasts or abdomen," Dr. Graham says. "That's how your skin would look now if you had protected it."

You can't erase the damage the sun has already done. But with sensible self-care, you can minimize its impact and keep your skin smooth, firm, and vibrant. Dr. Graham recommends these anti-aging tactics.

- Stay out of the sun, especially from 10:00 A.M. to 4:00 P.M., when the sun's rays are most intense.
- When you do head outdoors, wear sunscreen. Choose a product with a sun protection factor (SPF) of at least 15, and apply it at least 30 minutes before you go outside.
- Wear protective clothing. In general, tightly woven fabric, like that found in a heavyweight T-shirt, screens out the sun's rays better than loosely woven fabric.
- Wear sunglasses and a hat or visor.
- Avoid tanning beds.
- Keep your weight stable. Repeatedly losing and gaining causes skin to sag.
- Avoid cosmetics that clog the skin's hair follicles, causing blemishes. Look for products labeled "nonacnegenic" (won't provoke acne) and "noncomedogenic" (won't provoke blackheads and whiteheads).
- Remove makeup adequately and thoroughly.
- Use an abrasive sponge (like a loofah or Buf-Puf) to get rid of dead skin cells and open the skin's hair follicles. Keep the sponge away from the delicate area around your eyes.
- If you smoke, quit. Smoking depletes vitamin C from the skin, and repeatedly pursing your lips around a cigarette causes wrinkles around your mouth.

Certain nutritional supplements can also help keep your skin healthy and young-looking. "I've started taking supplements myself for my skin," Dr. Graham says. "I used to think I didn't need to because I never spent a lot of time in the sun. But my skin looks better, and I feel better. I've become a believer." She suggests the following nutrition prescription.

- 5,000 international units (IU) of vitamin A daily. A deficiency of vitamin A can leave skin rough and scaly.
- 500 milligrams of vitamin C daily. Vitamin C supports the formation of collagen, the connective tissue that gives skin its structure and tone.
- 400 IU of vitamin E daily. An antioxidant, vitamin E helps protect the skin against sun damage.
- 200 micrograms of selenium daily. People with low levels of selenium appear most prone to skin cancer.

Age Spots

Don't let their name fool you: Age spots have nothing to do with age. Rather, these flat, brown patches result from overexposure to the sun.

You can easily prevent age spots just by slathering on sunscreen before heading outdoors. Unfortunately, truly protective sunscreen products didn't appear on the market until the early 1980s. So anyone born before then is likely to develop age spots.

You can take steps to fade existing spots and discourage new spots from forming. Here's what to do.

Make 'em fade. Apply a fade cream that contains 2 percent hydroquinone. It will help diminish age spots, although they won't disappear completely. Follow the label directions carefully.

Discover AHAs. To lighten age spots and to even out your skin tone, apply a cream or lotion that contains alpha hydroxy acids (AHAs). These natural acids strip away dead skin cells and prompt the growth of fresh, new cells.

Choose a 5 percent AHA preparation, and, when applying, be careful to avoid your eyelids.

Wash your hands after handling food. Celery, limes, and some other foods contain psoralens, chemicals that can cause a sunburnlike reaction in the skin when exposed to sunlight. The affected skin eventually blisters and heals with hyperpigmentation (darker skin), which can persist for weeks to months.

Monitor medicines. Certain drugs make your skin more sensitive to sunlight, so you are more likely to develop age spots. Among the offenders are Retin-A, used for acne and wrinkles; antibiotics such as tetracycline; and blood pressure and diabetes medications.

Blemishes

Blemishes don't confine themselves to teenage faces. If conditions are right, they intrude on adult complexions too.

Blemishes seem to come and go with hormonal fluctuations. Don't believe those stories that blemishes come from eating greasy foods or having poor hygiene. Such claims are groundless. In fact, washing too often can irritate the skin and aggravate acne.

Products containing benzoyl peroxide or salicylic acid dry out blemishes so that they go away faster. But benzoyl peroxide, in particular, can irritate the skin. To combat breakouts naturally, try these self-care measures.

Put your washcloth away. For daily care, wash your face (including underneath your chin) with a pH-balanced sensitive-skin cleanser and warm water. Use your hands, rather than a washcloth, to avoid aggravating inflammation. Rinse thoroughly. Repeat no more than twice a day.

Take a Good Look at Your Back

Though most moles are benign (noncancerous), some have the potential to develop into cancer, especially when they are irregular in shape and color.

While only a trained dermatologist can tell them apart, it is a good idea to check yourself for certain changes in moles so you can quickly identify changes that warrant attention. Early treatment boosts the rate of success and reduces your risk of having skin cancer spread. You need to look for new moles *and* check pre existing ones for changes.

You can give your back a checkup by using a hand-held mirror and a full-length mirror or by enlisting the aid of your spouse or a friend, says Jean Bolognia, M.D., director of the Pigmented Lesion Clinic at the Yale University School of Medicine.

When checking moles, think A-B-C-D.

A (asymmetry). Normal moles are symmetrical—if you draw a line down the middle of them, the halves match. Melanomas have halves that don't match.

B (border). Normal moles have smooth, regular borders. Melanomas have blurred, irregular ones.

C (color). Normal moles have uniform coloring. Melanomas may have a variety of colors: red, black, brown, tan, and white.

D (diameter). A normal mole is no bigger than the circumference of a pencil eraser. Most melanomas have a larger diameter.

If you notice any of these variations, make an appointment to see your doctor as soon as possible.

Come clean with steam. A facial steam bath made with elder flowers, yarrow, and chamomile helps remove the dirt and pus that clog pores. Put a handful of each of the dried herbs in a large pot, and cover with 1 to 2 quarts of water. Bring to a slow, gentle simmer. Remove the pot from the stove and set it where you can lean over it. Drape a towel over your head, creating a tent over the pot. Soak in the steam for up to 15 minutes.

Yield to yarrow's benefits. Put 1 ounce of dried yarrow in a quart jar. Fill the jar with boiling water, then cover and allow to steep overnight. In the morning, strain out the yarrow and store the liquid in a plastic bottle. Dampen a washcloth with the liquid and gently pat it on your face twice daily, morning and evening. Yarrow is a powerful herbal antiseptic.

Fight zits with B_6. Vitamin B_6 helps control breakouts, especially in women whose acne worsens during their menstrual cycles. You can safely take up to 50 milligrams a day.

Bruises

Like a cut, a bruise involves bleeding. With a bruise, though, the bleeding occurs beneath the surface of the skin, when an accidental encounter with something hard breaks blood vessels. Blood leaks out, producing telltale discoloration as well as swelling and soreness.

In general, the farther down a bruise is located on your body, the longer it takes to heal. A leg bruise can hang around for up to a month, primarily because leg vessels have greater blood pressure.

To minimize discoloration and encourage speedy healing, follow this advice.

Use ice first. Applying ice right after the initial bump can limit the size and severity of a bruise. Wrap the ice in a towel, elevate the bruised area, and then ice the bruise for 20 minutes.

Save heat for later. Applying heat to a bruise dilates blood vessels in the area so they can clear away blood cells and fluid. Wait at least 24 hours after the initial bump so that the bruise is fully developed. Then soak a washcloth in comfortably hot water and lay it over the bruise for 20 minutes. Repeat three times a day.

Opt for Arnica. A homeopathic remedy, Arnica has long been used to treat bruises, although no one knows why it works. Apply the cream, ointment, or oil once a day for 2 to 3 days. Avoid using it on broken skin since it can cause a rash.

Rub in vitamin K. In cream form, vitamin K helps the body break down blood at the bruise site and reabsorb it. Apply the cream as soon as possible after the bruise occurs, and repeat twice a day until the bruise fades.

Chafing

When body parts rub against each other, they create friction. Friction, in turn, scrapes away skin cells. If you remove enough skin cells in this manner, the body's immune system jumps into action. The affected skin becomes raw, red, and inflamed—all classic signs of chafing.

If chafing is severe, bacteria, fungi, and other microorganisms that normally reside on the surface of the skin can find their way under the skin. There, they can cause infection.

Fortunately, chafing never has to go that far, if you take care of the irritated skin early on. Here's how.

Wash and dry. If a workout leaves your skin sweaty and raw, jump into the shower and let the water run over the chafed area. Use an antibacterial soap to destroy bacteria, yeast, and fungi. Rinse thoroughly to wash away soap residue, which can aggravate chafing. Then set your blow-dryer on low, and dry the chafed skin.

Soften after your shower. If your skin is raw but not bloody, apply moisturizer after bathing. The moisturizer traps water on your skin, preventing further drying.

The Right Way to Wax

Waxing is the best way to remove hair from your bikini line as well as from your upper lip, says Alla Zelikovsky, an aesthetician (beauty expert) at the Elizabeth Arden Red Door Salon in New York City. And it needn't be messy, time-consuming, or painful. Here's her step-by-step technique.

Bikini Area

1. Any brand of wax is fine, but Zelikovsky recommends beeswax (available in health food stores). It's lighter than other waxes, so the waxing goes faster and is not as messy or painful.
2. In a double boiler, heat the wax until most, but not all, has melted. Melting all of it will make the wax thin, sticky, and hard to work with.
3. Sprinkle a little talcum powder over the area to be waxed. It will cut the oil on your skin, which can keep wax from adhering. It will also make the hair stand up.
4. Drop a pearl-size drop of wax on your wrist or in your palm. If it is too hot, wait.
5. Using the backside of a teaspoon, apply using "up" strokes, *against* the direction of hair growth. Using down strokes will make the wax difficult and painful to remove. Wax no more than a 2-inch strip of hair at a time and don't apply the wax too thickly. Finally, wax one bikini line at a time.

Try tea tree oil. This essential oil, sold in health food stores, protects chafed skin from infection and speeds healing. Soak a cotton ball in water, apply a few drops of the oil to the cotton, and then press the cotton against the chafed area. Repeat several times a day until your skin improves.

6. Slather the freshly waxed area with a lotion formulated with the herb chamomile, available in health food stores. "Chamomile calms the skin," says Zelikovsky.
7. No matter what you do, wax will cling to your skin, says Zelikovsky. Start to remove the wax after it has hardened slightly but while it is still a little supple. Slather the area with an oily cold cream and pull off as much as you can in the direction it was applied (against the growth).
8. Wait for regrowth. Never shave your bikini line between waxings. "Shaving makes the hair like wire," says Zelikovsky.

Upper Lip Area

1. Follow steps 1 through 4 above.
2. Apply the wax in five separate "pieces," waxing from the corners of your mouth, in. Wax the left side of your mouth, then the right. Next, wax the left middle part of the lip line, then the right. Last, wax the area directly under your nose. To remove, pull the wax up, not down. Removing that last piece of wax can bring tears to your eyes. To make it less painful, form an extra ball of warm wax, press it to the waxed area, and pull.
3. To minimize redness and swelling, wipe the area with an antiseptic and pat with ice.

Note: If you have very sensitive skin, first test the oil by placing a drop on a clean area of arm skin. If you don't experience any irritation within 24 hours, go ahead and use the oil.

Dry Skin

Dry, chapped, cracked skin won't protect you from viruses and infections as well as it should. So keeping it hydrated is essential. It is also quite easy to do, as these tips demonstrate.

Moisturize with milk. Pour cold milk into a bowl or basin, then dip a washcloth or a piece of gauze in the milk and hold it against the affected skin for 5 minutes. Milk soothes dry skin and has anti-inflammatory properties to relieve itching.

Moisturize with mineral oil. Plain old mineral oil traps moisture in the skin, helping it stay hydrated.

Rehydrate at bedtime. Before going to bed, soak in a lukewarm bath almost to the point where your fingertips shrivel like prunes—your skin will be fully hydrated. Get out of the tub, pat yourself semidry, and apply a thick layer of shortening to the affected skin. Slip into an old pair of pajamas and climb into bed.

Cleanse gently. For your daily shower or bath, use lukewarm water and very mild soap. If your skin is extremely dry, avoid strong antibacterial soaps, which tend to dry skin.

Ingrown Hair

If you shave too close, you can nick the top of a hair follicle, causing it to become partially obstructed. The hair inside then grows at an angle, eventually piercing the side of the follicle and burying itself in your skin. The skin becomes inflamed and produces a tiny red bump, the familiar mark of an ingrown hair.

An ingrown hair can also occur when an individual hair grows straight out of its follicle, then curls down and reenters the follicle.

Whatever the cause, an ingrown hair usually heals on its own within 2 weeks. To speed healing and prevent a recurrence, follow this advice.

Soothe with soap. Wash the area around the ingrown hair twice each day with an antibacterial soap. Follow up with a dab of benzoyl peroxide cream, found at drugstores. This helps reduce the inflammation.

Change blades regularly. If an ingrown hair has become infected, change your razor blade each time you shave until the hair heals. Otherwise, it could become reinfected.

Shield your skin. When shaving, protect hair follicles from nicks by creating a moisture barrier between your skin and the blade. A mild soap will do the job, although you can also use a shaving foam or gel.

Oily Skin

Everyone's skin has a coating of oil, or sebum, to keep out dirt and make skin soft and supple. Sometimes the oil becomes too thick, thanks to overproductive sebaceous glands.

Like dry skin, oily skin becomes a problem only when it isn't properly cared for. You can minimize the sheen and reduce the likelihood of breakouts by following this advice.

Buy the right bar. To wash your face, use a soap made with glycerin, cucumber, witch hazel, or citrus acids. These natural ingredients keep oily skin healthy.

Lather up less. Washing your face too often may stimulate your skin to produce *more* oil. Limit yourself to three times a day.

Try a natural toner. After washing your face, apply witch hazel, using a cotton ball. Witch hazel cleans soap residue and reduces the amount of oil on your skin.

Fight oil with (essential) oil. Add two drops of lemongrass essential oil to 1 tablespoon of a carrier oil such as apricot kernel, flaxseed, or hazelnut (available in health food stores). With a cotton ball or your clean fingers, gently apply the mixture to your face after every cleansing. Lemongrass helps degrease the skin and regulates overactive sebaceous glands, but keep it away from your eyes.

Rashes

Think of a rash as your body's built-in distress signal. That red, itchy patch of skin may be telling you that you have come into contact with an irritant such as a harsh detergent, poison ivy, or even rubber. Or it may be a signal that you are having an allergic reaction to a food or a medication. Or it may be a sign of illness.

Depending on its cause, a rash may take a week or longer to heal. You can minimize itching and discomfort, in the meantime, with these self-care measures. (If your rash gets worse after a day or two or if it is accompanied by fever, headache, joint pain, or difficulty breathing, see your doctor right away.)

Sit in soda. Pour ½ cup of baking soda into a tub full of lukewarm water, then climb in for a 15-minute soak. You could also make a paste from a spoonful of baking soda mixed with a little water and dab that on your rash to soothe your skin. Baking soda helps relieve itching.

Make a milk compress. Combine one part milk and one part water, then soak a washcloth in the mixture and lay it over the rash. Milk's anti-inflammatory properties reduce itching. Remember to rinse off afterward.

Consider coal tar. Look in your drugstore for oils and gels made with coal tar, a potent anti-itch ingredient. Rub the oil or gel onto the affected skin, following the label directions. Because coal tar can stain, your best bet is to apply it at bedtime, then slip into old pajamas and sleep on old sheets.

Cool with cornstarch. Ordinary cornstarch can be quite soothing on a rash. Just sprinkle some on the affected skin.

Scarring

For folks who have one, a scar usually serves as a visible reminder of something they'd just as soon forget—a too-close encounter with a paring knife, a fall off a bicycle, a chance step onto a piece of glass. Injuries like these can damage the deepest layer of skin, called the dermis. When that happens, the body produces new tissue to repair the wound, and a scar forms. Scarring can also follow a serious case of adolescent acne or a surgical incision.

Whether you want to prevent scarring or fade an existing scar, these measures can help.

Take supplemental C. While your skin is on the mend, take 250 milligrams of vitamin C twice each day—once in the morning, once in the evening. Vitamin C speeds wound healing.

Massage the skin. Once the skin has healed, firmly massage the area once or twice a day for 2 months. Putting pressure on the injury supports the wound-healing process, making the scar less prominent.

Butter it up. For an existing scar, apply cocoa butter lotion or cream every day. The cocoa butter keeps the scar from becoming more prominent.

Sensitive Skin

If you have sensitive skin, certain substances can make your skin itch, burn, sting, or break out in a red, swollen rash or tiny blisters. Among the common culprits are ingredients in skin-care products, cosmetics, and household cleaners.

Sometimes what looks like a run-of-the-mill skin irritation is actually an allergic reaction. You can find out whether you have an allergy by asking your dermatologist to do a skin-patch test.

Whatever the cause of your sensitive skin, you can reduce your chances of a flare-up by following this skin-care routine.

Cut your bath time. Keep your baths or showers short. Use cool or lukewarm water and a mild, fragrance- and preservative-free cleanser. Be sure to thoroughly rinse your skin to remove any cleanser residue, then pat dry.

Stick with hypoallergenic products. Hypoallergenic products contain fewer skin-irritating fragrances and preservatives than "regular" products.

Leave scents alone. Fragrance is among the most common skin irritant. Products labeled "unscented" or "fragrance-free" may actually contain fragrance to mask the odors of other ingredients. So read labels and steer clear of products that use words such as *fragrance*, *perfume*, and *aromatherapy* or that contain any of the botanicals, including chamomile, rosewood, lavender, lemon, and rosemary.

Check for formaldehyde. Formaldehyde, another common skin irritant, is found in shampoos, makeup, and many skin-care products. But you probably won't see it listed as an ingredient. Instead, read labels for quaternium #15, DMDM hydantoin, imidazolidinyl urea, diazolidinyl urea, or Bronopol—chemical additives that release formaldehyde over time.

Spider Veins

At least 40 percent of women develop spider veins—networks of tiny red, blue, or purple blood vessels that appear on the upper thighs, behind the knees, and on the feet. They can be caused by a superficial injury, such as being hit by a tennis ball or being jumped on by a pet. They are also quite common during pregnancy.

Spider veins may be unsightly, but they seldom cause the pain and swelling associated with varicose veins. You can have them removed by laser or injection. If you prefer to go the natural route, doctors suggest these strategies.

Have a bowl of berries. Fruits like blueberries, blackberries, cherries, and raspberries supply bioflavonoids, natural compounds that help strengthen blood vessels. The darker the fruit, the more bioflavonoids it contains.

Don't peel away the pith. Pith, the white membrane in citrus fruits such as oranges and grapefruit, provides a healthy dose of bioflavonoids as well.

Go for ginkgo. The herb ginkgo helps strengthen the tissues that form vein walls. Look for a 50:1 extract, which will be specified on the label. Take 40 milligrams three times a day until your spider veins are diminished.

Stretch Marks

Most women associate stretch marks with pregnancy. But the scarlike lesions can result from weight gain, exercises that bulk up the muscles—anything that makes the skin's elastic tissue stretch and tear. They have also been linked to prolonged use of high-potency cortisone creams and other corticosteroid medications, which cause the skin to become thin.

For stretch marks, prevention is the best medicine. Once you have them, all the cocoa butter, olive oil, and vitamin E gel in the world won't make them disappear. The best you can do is to minimize their appearance. Here's how.

Do the right moves. The following exercises can firm the areas with stretch marks, making the lesions less visible. To start, do 8 to 10 repetitions of each exercise three times a week. Gradually work your way up to 20 reps three times a week.

To firm your hips and legs: Lie on the floor on your side with your thighs together, top leg straight and bottom leg bent at the knee. Extend the arm that's closest to the floor over your head and rest your head on your arm. Put your other hand flat on the floor in front of your waist. Keeping your top leg straight and your toes pointed straight ahead, slowly raise your top leg from hip to toe about 1 foot off the ground, then slowly lower it back to the floor. Don't just jerk your leg up in the air and let it fall back down. Instead, raise and lower your leg in a slow, controlled motion. Do all of your repetitions before switching legs.

To firm your inner thighs: Lie on your side, supporting your head with your hand. Keep your bottom leg straight. Bending the top leg, place your foot flat on the floor in front of your bottom leg. Try to raise the bottom leg about 6 inches, then lower it. Do all of your repetitions before switching legs.

To firm your bottom: Lie facedown on the floor with a pillow under your hips. Turn your head to one side and rest your cheek on your clasped hands. Raise one leg off the floor, heel first, 3 to 6 inches, then lower it. Repeat with your other leg, then continue alternating legs.

Moms-to-be, moisturize. If you are pregnant, apply moisturizer to your abdomen twice a day. Your skin's elastic tissue stretches more and tears less when it is moisturized, so stretch marks are less likely to form.

Sunburn

Fair-skinned blondes and redheads tend to burn more easily than dark-skinned brunettes. Likewise, people taking certain medications, including birth control pills and estrogen replacement pills, can become more sensitive to the sun.

If you find yourself nursing a sunburn, the following tips can help relieve the redness and discomfort. (Be sure to see your doctor if you experience severe pain, blistering, or excessive swelling.)

Soak in oatmeal. To relieve the itchiness of dried, sunburned skin, add 1 cup of colloidal oatmeal (sold in drugstores) to a tub full of cool water. Then soak for 15 minutes.

Apply an aloe/lavender combination. Squeeze the gel from a whole aloe leaf and add one or two drops of lavender essential oil. Lightly apply the gel to sunburned skin. Repeat two or three times a day until the pain subsides. This powerful antiseptic and antibacterial formula can speed the healing process.

Relieve pain with plantain. An herbal wash made from plantain leaves may take away the sting of sunburn. You can buy the dried leaves in some health food stores. Grind up a few leaves, place them in a cup of boiling water, and steep for a few minutes. When the liquid cools, pour or splash it onto the sunburned skin. You can use the wash once or twice a day. Do not confuse the plant plantain with the banana-like fruit of the same name.

Ease the pain with E. Take 400 IU of vitamin E every 4 hours (while awake) for one day, starting immediately after getting a sunburn. The d-alpha-tocopherol form of the vitamin works best. Studies have shown it contains an amino acid that reduces skin damage caused by sunburn.

Varicose Veins

Veins become varicose, or swollen, when the valves lining the vein walls fail to do their job. Normally, these valves prevent blood from flowing backward when it is making a return trip to the heart. A valve opens, the blood goes through, and the valve closes. But if that valve malfunctions, it allows the blood to reverse direction and pool in the vein. Eventually, the pressure created by the pooled blood stretches the vein wall. That's when the vein becomes visible on the surface of the skin.

Why do some people get varicose veins while others don't? It's genetics, mostly. If your mother or father has varicose veins, you are likely to have them too. Your risk increases if you are overweight or you stand for 6 or more hours a day.

Pregnancy can also contribute to the development of varicose veins. The hormonal changes that occur during pregnancy allow the veins to stretch to accommodate extra bloodflow. And the weight of the fetus can interfere with bloodflow and put greater pressure on the leg veins, especially during the third trimester.

Fortunately, you don't have to put up with unsightly veins that make your legs feel tired and heavy. These strategies can minimize your discomfort and keep varicose veins from worsening.

Comfort with a compress. Put ½ to 1 cup of distilled witch hazel in a bowl and refrigerate it for at least 1 hour. Then add six drops of cypress essential oil, one drop of lemon essential oil, and one drop of bergamot essential oil. Soak a cloth in the witch hazel solution, then lay the cloth over the varicose vein for 15 minutes. While applying the compress, elevate your feet on a few pillows to support circulation. Both the witch hazel and the essential oils have an astringent effect—they shrink small blood vessels near the surface of the skin, temporarily reducing swelling.

Try aescin. In one study, taking 50 milligrams of aescin (the extract from the dried seeds of the horse chestnut plant) twice a day for 12 weeks reduced the lower-leg swelling associated with varicose veins by 25 percent. Aescin is available at health food stores.

Get your fill of roughage. Every day, eat at least 25 grams (the Daily Value) of fiber. A fiber-rich diet featuring whole grains, fruits, and vegetables helps prevent constipation by making stool easier to pass. When you strain to move your bowels, you create pressure in your abdomen that can block the flow of blood to your legs. Over time, the increased pressure may weaken the walls of the veins in your legs.

Stock up on C. Your body uses vitamin C to build collagen and elastin, connective tissues that help strengthen vein walls. Take 500 milligrams twice a day.

Move your legs. Even while you are sitting, you can do exercises to keep the blood in your legs circulating. Here's one to try. Flex your feet, lifting your toes while keeping your heels down, as though you were pumping a piano pedal. Continue for a minute or two, then repeat every hour.

Wrinkles

Unprotected sun exposure is the leading cause of wrinkles. It wreaks havoc on the skin by breaking down collagen and elastin, two connective tissues that give skin its structure and tone.

Fortunately, skin—like the rest of the body—has the capacity to repair itself. You can take steps to diminish existing wrinkles and discourage new ones from appearing. Here's what dermatologists recommend.

Say yes to AHAs. Alpha hydroxy acids (AHAs) loosen and remove old, wrinkled cells to uncover the young, fresh cells underneath. And they plump the skin's surface, in essence filling in the "dents" that you see as wrinkles. Use an 8 percent AHA preparation on your face and neck twice a day—once in the morning and once at night. For the sensitive area around the eyes, use a fragrance-free 5 percent AHA eye cream and avoid getting it into your eyes or on your eyelashes. If you do, thoroughly rinse the affected eye with cold water.

Moisturize in the morning. Plumping the skin with moisturizer can help hide wrinkles. But most people apply moisturizer before bed, so their appearance is improved for only 4 to 6 hours while they sleep. You are better off moisturizing first thing in the morning.

Smooth on topical vitamin C. Unlike AHAs, which reverse skin damage by speeding up the exfoliation process, vitamin C might help prevent damage in the first place. As an antioxidant, vitamin C protects against wrinkles by fighting off free radicals, unstable molecules that form when the skin is exposed to sunlight and ultraviolet radiation and that harm healthy cells and contribute to skin damage.

Applying vitamin C directly to the skin can help prevent depletion of the nutrient when you spend a lot of time in the sun. One topical vitamin C product is Cellex-C. It's a 10 percent vitamin C solution that is available without a prescription from dermatologists and licensed aestheticians.

Great Hair Secrets

The way you wear your hair helps define you as a person. There is nothing about your looks that can so dramatically change your image. This is why so many of us fret so over our hair. We perm it, straighten it, tease it, roll it, iron it, primp it, color it, and frizz it. Bad hair day? Yes, we've all been there.

Maybe it's time to relax a little. There is a limit to what we can do with our hair because the course of our hair—the type, texture, and color—was genetically determined at conception, notes Patricia Farris, M.D., clinical assistant professor of dermatology at Tulane University School of Medicine in New Orleans.

"Unfortunately, most women don't realize the damage that overprocessing can do to their hair," says Dr. Farris. "Even blow-drying or using any heated styling appliance makes hair dry, brittle, and prone to breakage over time."

The effects of overprocessing are compounded by the fact that hair naturally dries out with age. "As you get older, your skin's sebaceous glands don't function as efficiently," Dr. Farris explains. "Without the sebum produced by these glands to provide lubrication, your scalp and hair become drier." Your hair may become thinner, too, especially after menopause.

Even if your hair has endured years of harsh treatments, you can take steps to repair any existing damage and restore life and luster. Here's what you can do to make your hair look its natural best.

Bad Hair Days

For those days when you can't get your hair headed in the right direction, here's what to do.

Go wrong. Wet your comb and run it through your hair in the direction opposite your usual style. Repeat a few times, then retrain your hair to go in the right direction.

Be mist-ifying. Fill a misting bottle (like the ones used to spray plants) with clean water. Then mist your hair, put some gel on it, and run a comb through it. No matter what gel you choose, start with less than the amount that the label instructions suggest.

Give curls a boost. Use a curling iron to restore bounce and body to curly or wavy hair. To prevent split ends, first cool the iron by rolling it in a wet towel. If your hair still goes limp, try boosting the curl with a little spray.

Subdue static. For flyaway hair, spray on a thermal styling conditioner right after shampooing and conditioning. Blow-dry your hair, using the lowest setting and holding the dryer 6 to 8 inches from your head. Or set your hair with Velcro rollers, then blow-dry.

Dandruff

Human skin is constantly recreating itself. The cells migrate to the surface, then slough off. Usually, this process takes about 21 days. Sometimes, though, the cells turn around in half the time and end up forming clumps on your scalp. In no time, you're Snow White.

Here's what you can do to dwarf the problem.

Lather your locks daily. Shampooing cleans dead skin cells from your scalp. So the more you do it, the better you'll control your dandruff.

Use the right shampoo. Choose a dandruff shampoo made with tar, selenium, or zinc pyrithione. These ingredients remove scaly patches from your scalp and relieve itching.

Double up. When washing your hair with a dandruff shampoo, lather once and rinse well. Lather again, this time really rubbing your scalp. Then let the shampoo sit for at least 5 minutes to give the active ingredient a chance to work. Rinse thoroughly.

Pull a switcheroo. Use your dandruff shampoo every day for 2 weeks. Then cut back to every other day, alternating it with a gentle nonmedicated shampoo. This protects your hair against the drying effects of the chemicals in dandruff shampoo. (If you don't notice any improvement in the first 2 weeks of using a dandruff shampoo, you may have a condition other than dandruff. See your doctor.)

Skip the conditioner. Heavy after-shampoo conditioners make dandruff worse. So if your hair becomes dry from using a non-tar-based dandruff shampoo, alternate it with a tar-based shampoo. Tar leaves hair soft and tangle-free.

Put moisture back. Drinking at least eight 8-ounce glasses of water a day moisturizes your scalp from the inside out. Fruits and vegetables also help you stay hydrated.

Dry Hair

In healthy hair, the cells that make up each strand's outer layer, called the cuticle, overlap like shingles on a roof. If the cells are roughed up or chipped away, the strand loses moisture and doesn't reflect light as it should. So hair not only feels dry but looks dry too.

With a few simple changes in your hair-care routine, you can repair the damage that leads to dry hair.

Be picky about shampoo. Look for a shampoo that contains aloe, glycerin, honey, amino acids, or natural oils. All of these substances moisturize hair. Steer clear of products that combine shampoo and conditioner; they neither clean nor condition well.

Get into condition. After shampooing, apply an instant conditioner that has been formulated for dry hair. Such a product protects against damage from drying and styling.

Moisturize with essential oils. If you can't find a commercial conditioner that you like, make your own. Add six drops each of lavender, bay, and sandalwood essential oils (available in health food stores) to ¾ cup of warm sesame or soy oil. Part your hair into 1-inch sections and apply the oil blend to your scalp with a wad of cotton. Wrap your head in a towel and wait 15 minutes. Then uncover your hair and shampoo twice.

Dry wisely. Whenever possible, use only a towel to pat or gently squeeze water from your hair. If you must use a blow-dryer, apply a thermal styling conditioner to protect your hair. Set the dryer on high to remove residual water, then switch to low for styling. Hold the dryer at least 6 to 8 inches from your hair at all times.

Outsmart the sun. To prevent sun damage, mist your hair with a styling product that contains sunscreen or a sun filter such as octyl-dimethyl PABA. And wear a lightweight, tightly woven hat with a wide brim.

Do a pre-swim prep. Before swimming in a chlorinated pool, apply an instant conditioner to your hair, and slip on a swim cap. Afterward, thoroughly rinse your hair, then wash it as usual.

FOLK REMEDY: DOES IT WORK?

Beer for Shiny Hair

Damage to the outer layer of the hair shaft (the cuticle) makes hair lose its shine. The cuticle is lined with scales that resemble shingles on a rooftop. When the scales lie flat, they reflect light. Sun exposure, overbrushing, and chemical assaults on your hair loosen the shingles, so they curl upward and make hair look dull.

The protein found in beer can fill in the irregular surface between the scales, causing a smoother appearance and more shine, says Leslie Baumann, M.D., director and assistant professor of cosmetic dermatology at the University of Miami. For the best results, soak your hair thoroughly with the beer, then rinse. Be sure to use beer that's fresh and still foaming because the proteins necessary to make the head on the beer are the same ones that add shine to hair. Stale beer has no head because these proteins have already been broken down. And just as with any conditioner, beer's shining effect lasts only until the next washing.

Recommendation: Worth a Try

Frizzies

If the frizzies have rendered your mane unmanageable, you can bring them under control. The key is to get your hair in top condition. Start with these strategies.

Massage, don't scrub. Choose a shampoo formulated for dry or damaged hair. Massage it onto your scalp with your fingertips, then gently work it through your hair with your fingers. Leave your hair hanging down as you wash it, rather than bunching it on top of your head, which causes breakage.

Gently detangle. After shampooing, work a quarter-size dollop of detangling conditioner through your hair. (Avoid products that are heavy, waxy, or silicone-based.) Gently run a wide-toothed comb through your hair, proceeding in small sections from the ends toward your scalp. Stop when you're about an inch from your scalp. Leave the detangler on for 2 to 3 minutes so that your hair has a chance to absorb the moisture. Then rinse, leaving a little of the detangler in.

Restore hair from the inside. A good deep conditioner fills hair shafts with protein so that hair repels moisture better. Look for a product that contains wheat germ or soybean protein. Apply it twice a month to start, then cut back to once a month as your hair improves. (If you color your hair, avoid using hot-oil treatments and other heated deep conditioners for at least 10 days afterward. Otherwise, the color will fade or turn brassy.)

Add gel. Molding gel seals out excessive moisture and protects against environmental elements. Work the gel into sections of wet hair, starting at the nape of your neck and moving up toward the center of your head. Repeat, each time sliding your fingers closer to your ears. Finish with the forehead and hairline area.

Put away the blow-dryer. After shampooing and conditioning, squeeze excess water from your hair, using a towel. Then allow your hair to air-dry.

Gray Hair

Graying is hereditary, and there's no avoiding it. Everyone eventually goes gray as individual hair follicles stop producing pigment.

Surprisingly, only about one-third of all women opt for the cover-up. The rest let nature make the choice. But even Mother Nature has some secrets to help give gray hair a youthful sheen.

Rinse with sage or rosemary. To gently darken brown or black hair that's showing signs of gray, use a rinse made from sage or rosemary. Add between 2 teaspoons and 1 tablespoon of either dried herb to a cup of boiling water. Let the liquid cool to a comfortable temperature, strain, and pour it over your hair after shampooing. Don't rinse it out. Repeat each time you wash your hair until you've covered the gray.

Add nettle and walnut to the mix. For auburn, brown, or medium to dark gray hair, use a coloring made with nettle and black walnut hulls (available at health food stores or by mail-order catalogs). To prepare the coloring, boil 8 cups of water and add ¼ cup each of dried sage, rosemary, and nettle; ½ cup of black walnut hulls; and two black tea bags. Allow the mixture to steep for 3 hours, then strain and add 2 teaspoons of sweet almond or olive oil. Keep the mixture refrigerated until you're ready to use it. After you wash and rinse your hair, slip on a pair of rubber gloves and work ½ cup of the mixture through your hair, being careful not to get it on your forehead, neck, and temples. Wait a minute or so before towel-drying your hair. Use a dark towel so that the stains won't show.

Oily Hair

The term *oily hair* is something of a misnomer. The oil comes not from your hair but from your scalp. Like the rest of your skin, your scalp has sebaceous glands. They secrete sebum, a mixture of fatty acids that keep your scalp from drying out. In some people, the sebaceous glands churn out so much sebum that each hair shaft becomes slickly coated and weighted down. Hair appears greasy, flat, and lifeless.

Sebum production is regulated by hormones. Women who have oily hair often find that the problem literally dries up after they go through menopause, when their hormone levels decline. In the meantime, you can control greasiness by following this advice.

Wash in the morning. You work up a sweat while you sleep. So by morning, even hair shampooed just before bedtime looks oily and matted.

Stir up your own shampoo. Add four drops of rosemary essential oil and four drops of lavender essential oil to ¼ cup of any unscented shampoo. Shake to mix well, then use a quarter-size dollop to wash your hair. Rosemary and lavender tone your scalp and add shine. The essential oils are available in health food stores and bath-and-beauty shops.

Trade off. Alternate your regular shampoo with a clarifying shampoo, which removes oil from the hair shaft as well as from your scalp. Check labels for a product that is high in cleaning agents such as sodium lauryl sulfate and low in conditioning agents such as lanolin.

Rinse with vinegar. Vinegar reduces soap and hard-water residues to make your hair soft and shiny. Mix 1 cup of vinegar with 1 cup of water, then pour the solution over your hair as a final rinse. Vinegar's aroma quickly fades.

Curtail conditioning. Most conditioners and styling products contain ingredients that weigh hair down, which is the last thing you need if your hair is oily.

Cut back on brushing. The more you brush, the more you spread oil from your scalp to your hair.

Split Ends

What with blow-dryers, curling irons, and other heated styling appliances, there is no end to the times we end up with split ends. The intense temperature causes hair strands to crack at the tip and split up the shaft.

Keeping up with your haircuts is the easiest way to make split ends disappear. Just make sure that the stylist is using sharp scissors. Dull scissors can actually cause split ends. If you tend to have long spells between cuts, here's what to do.

Get in the thick of things. Look for a shampoo and a conditioner that contain waxes or other thickening agents.

Allow hair to air-dry. The intense heat from blow-drying causes split ends.

Turn down the temp. If you must use a blow-dryer or another heated appliance, first spray your damp hair with a thermal styling conditioner. Then set the appliance on the lowest setting to minimize heat damage.

Thinning

Everyone sheds between 50 and 100 hairs per day. The average hair has a life span of 3 to 6 years, entering a resting stage of about 3 months before falling out. Then a new hair sprouts in its place from the same roots.

Sometimes, though, the hair growth cycle gets messed up, causing hundreds of hairs to fall out per day. In women, hormonal changes brought on by pregnancy, menopause, and the use of oral contraceptives can alter hair-growing conditions. So can rapid weight loss, iron deficiency, serious illness, and extreme physical stress (such as childbirth).

Some women even have a genetic predisposition to hair loss, just as some men do. It can come from either parent.

If you seem to be losing more hair than normal, see your doctor. She can examine you for an underlying medical problem and prescribe proper treatment. Then use these measures to care for your remaining hair and discourage more loss.

Baby your mane. Wash your hair with a baby shampoo, lathering up only once and rubbing your scalp gently.

After rinsing, spray your hair with a detangling conditioner.

Pull the plug. Allow your hair to dry naturally whenever possible. If you must use a blow-dryer, set it on low.

Wait while wet. Wait until your hair is completely dry before combing or brushing. Otherwise, it can stretch and break. And never tease your hair, which also causes breakage.

Get more B_6. Vitamin B_6 seems to slow the rate of hair loss in some people. Take 100 milligrams a day in supplement form.

Mine for iron. Iron deficiency can contribute to hair loss, so eat one to two servings of iron-rich foods every day. Good sources of the mineral include lean red meat, Cream of Wheat cereal, tofu, and broccoli.

Put protein on your plate. Without adequate protein, your body can't make new hair to replace what has fallen out. So eat two 3-to-4-ounce servings of chicken, fish, or other lean protein every day.

Sweet Relief for Feet

If you happen to visit a podiatrist's office anytime soon, take a look around the waiting room while you're there. Chances are that women will outnumber men four to one.

That's because women have four times as many foot problems as men. And women account for 90 percent of all foot surgeries. Not that women's feet are any different from men's, structurally speaking. Women just seem to have a propensity for squeezing them into shoes that are too high, too pointy, and too tight.

"Women's footwear has long been designed for style, rather than function," observes Pamela Colman, D.P.M., director of health affairs at the American Podiatric Medical Association. "Almost every common foot problem that you can think of—blisters, corns, calluses—results from poorly shaped, poorly constructed, ill-fitting shoes."

Women over age 65 are especially prone to foot problems because they've worn pointed-toe high heels for most of their lives. They have 3½ times more calluses and corns and 13 times more bunions than men of the same age.

Shoe Sense

The easiest way to keep your feet out of the doctor's office is to wear sensible shoes. Thankfully, many of us are getting the message. "Maybe it's because athletic shoes are 'in' right now, but I've noticed that more women are choosing footwear more for comfort than for style," Dr. Colman says.

How can you be sure that you're getting the best shoes for your feet? Dr. Colman offers this brief buyer's guide.

- Shop for shoes in the latter part of the day, when your feet have swollen to their maximum.
- Have both feet measured for length and width. "It's not at all unusual to have one foot be a little longer than the other," Dr. Colman says. If you do, fit shoes to the longer foot.
- Always try shoes on. "Manufacturers use different lasts, or forms, to make shoes," Dr. Colman explains. "So even though your foot measures a size 6, you may not be a size 6 in every brand of shoe."
- Look for shoes made from breathable material, like leather or canvas.
- Avoid styles with pointy toes or with heels higher than 2 inches.
- Buy the pair that feels most comfortable when you try them on. Don't expect to break them in.

Buying the right shoes is crucial, but it's only part of the equation. Dr. Colman suggests adding these strategies to your foot-care routine.

- Get rid of worn-out shoes. How can you tell? Set them on a table or on another flat surface. If they're not perfectly level—if either shoe tilts in or out—they're no longer supporting your feet as they should be.

• Wear flip-flops, rather than walk barefoot. Otherwise, you are exposing your feet not just to viruses and fungi but also to foreign objects.

• After bathing, be sure to dry between your toes. This area is a haven for moisture-loving, disease-causing microorganisms.

• After bathing, massage your feet with a moisturizing lotion.

• When giving yourself a pedicure, cut your toenails straight across and then gently file the edges with an emery board. You'll minimize your chances of getting an ingrown toenail.

All the above strategies can help keep your feet healthy and problem-free. But if you are bothered by a specific foot problem, read on for expert-recommended tips.

Blisters

Combine shoes that don't fit properly with almost any activity that has you on your feet, and you'll probably end up with a blister.

Although painful, a blister serves an important purpose. The fluid sealed inside keeps the skin moist and helps it heal. Ideally, the blister should be left intact to protect the skin against infection. But if it does open, that's okay, as long as you take extra care to keep the wound clean.

To baby your unbroken blister and speed the healing process, follow this advice.

Alleviate pain with aloe. A popular remedy for burns, aloe also heals blisters, thanks to its anti-inflammatory and antibiotic properties. Just smear some gel on the blister and cover it with gauze or a sterile bandage.

Be blister-free with comfrey. The herb comfrey contains the compound allantoin, which can help heal wounds. You can buy comfrey cream in health food stores. Or you can make a poultice from the herb by following this recipe: Cut up a handful of dried comfrey leaves (available at health food stores), cover them with boiling water, and let steep for 10 minutes. Allow to cool, then strain the leaves from the water. Gently squeeze the leaves to remove any excess water. Put the moistened herb on a piece of gauze, and place the gauze on top of the blister with the leaves on top of the gauze. Cover with another piece of gauze, and secure in place with an elastic bandage for at least 20 minutes. Do this twice daily.

Feel relief with calendula. A combination of the herb calendula and vitamin E can speed the healing of blisters by reducing inflammation. Mix equal parts calendula oil and vitamin E oil and spread it on the blister. Calendula and vitamin E oil are available in drugstores and health food stores.

If you don't have vitamin E oil on hand, poke open a vitamin E capsule with a pin and squeeze out the capsule's contents.

Give it air. You want to protect the blistered area with a bandage while you're wearing shoes. But when you can, take off your shoes and bandage, and allow the blister to breathe. Air helps it heal faster.

Pop with precision. If a blister becomes too uncomfortable, go ahead and pop it—the right way. Sterilize a needle by holding it to a small flame. Make several small holes at the sides of the blister. (Don't prick the blister only once; it may quickly reseal.) Allow the liquid to flow out of the holes. Leave the top flap of skin in place to protect the wound. Apply an antibiotic liquid over the area and cover it with gauze to eliminate bacteria that could cause infection. Change the gauze twice a day. If you have diabetes, you should not attempt this without consulting with your doctor.

Bunions

Does your foot resemble a triangle, with the tip of your big toe or little toe angling inward and your joint jutting outward? If so, you have a bunion. And it probably hurts.

While shoes can aggravate bunions, they don't actually cause them. You inherit the shape of your feet from your ancestors.

Many people can live with the discomfort of bunions. But sometimes the pain becomes so severe that simple physical activity such as walking becomes difficult. In such cases, surgery may provide the only real relief.

That said, you can do a lot on your own to keep your foot comfortable and prevent a bunion from getting worse. Start with these strategies.

Put your bunion on ice. Your bunion may be inflamed if it feels hot and swollen. You can cool it down with an ice pack wrapped in a damp cloth. Apply it to your bunion for 10 to 15 minutes.

Pick pineapple. Pineapple contains the compound bromelain, which acts as an anti-inflammatory to reduce the swelling and pain associated with bunions. Simply wipe the inside of a small piece of the peel from a fresh pineapple directly over your bunion. Or take 250 to 500 milligrams of pure bromelain in capsule form three times a day. You can find the capsules in health food stores and in some drugstores.

Buy new shoes. Although a change of footwear won't get rid of bunions, it may make them less painful. Wear athletic shoes as often as you can. They provide excellent comfort and support for feet with bunions. If you must wear dress shoes, choose a pair that has heels no higher than 1½ inches.

Calluses

Like a blister, a callus results from the friction created when shoe rubs against skin.

The Price of Pretty Feet

The perfect pedicure—soft, smooth skin and painted toes—may look great in sandals. But once you fling them off, you'll be hop, hop, hopping across the sand to escape the heat of the burning sun.

While many women are willing to pay a pretty price for creams and lotions for pretty feet, the calluses they are buffing away are making their feet (especially when going shoeless) more vulnerable to aches and pain.

"Calluses are nothing more than thickened skin caused by excessive pressure on part of the foot," explains Ellen J. Sobel, D.P.M., Ph.D., associate professor in the division of orthopedic sciences at the New York College of Podiatric Medicine in New York City. "They're not especially attractive but may offer protection."

For example, if you frequently wear high-heeled shoes, calluses help cushion those parts of your feet that bear your body weight. The same is true if you have high arches, flat feet, or some other structural problem. For women

Generally, a callus will become a problem only when it grows big enough to become a source of pressure and discomfort. Still, if you have one, you'd probably like to see it disappear. These self-care measures can help.

Put pumice to work. Use a pumice stone, which is actually volcanic glass, to rub off the dead skin of the callus and reveal the smoother skin underneath. You can buy pumice stones in drugstores, beauty supply stores, and some health food stores.

To begin, soak your feet in plain lukewarm water for 5 to 10 minutes to soften the callus. Then gently who are on their feet all day, calluses are the cushions that keep their feet from aching.

What's more, while callus-removing products seem harmless enough, they can make matters worse if they're not used properly. "The patients I see usually leave them on too long," Dr. Sobel says. "They're only supposed to be left on overnight. They can burn the skin; it actually turns white."

Still, Dr. Sobel believes that callus-removing products have their place. "Provided they're applied according to the label directions, they can be especially effective for very thick calluses on the heels or under the metatarsals (the bones that connect the toes to the midfoot)," she says. "But really, if your callus doesn't cause any pain or discomfort, I'd recommend leaving it alone."

And if you have diabetes, never try to remove a callus on your own. The decreased sensitivity in your feet can make a minor problem much worse. See a podiatrist.

rub the stone back and forth across the callus. (If you have diabetes, decreased circulation, or decreased sensitivity, talk to your podiatrist before you attempt this.)

Let E do the healing. After rubbing the callus with a pumice stone, apply a vitamin E cream or oil. Vitamin E penetrates well and keeps the skin soft.

Use the correct lotion. Lotions made with urea can help prevent a hard callus by getting rid of dead skin and stopping its buildup. Look for them in drugstores and large supermarkets.

Corns

Corns form the same way calluses do, as layers of skin build up to protect points on the feet against constant rubbing by ill-fitting shoes. The main difference between the two is that corns sprout on top of or between toes, while calluses develop primarily on the heels and soles.

If a corn becomes thick enough to put pressure on nerves, it can hurt. But you don't have to live with the discomfort. Try these self-care strategies instead.

Change your lacing. If you have a corn on top of your toe, run the lace of your shoe from one bottom eyelet to the top eyelet on the opposite side. Weave the lace through the remaining eyelets, alternating from side to side. Tying your shoe in this way lifts the toebox, so your toes have more room.

Cushion the corn. To lessen the pain of a corn located between your toes, cover it with a tuft of lamb's wool, available in drugstores.

Rub in castor oil. Castor oil softens corns and makes them less painful and easier to file down with a pumice stone. Massage your feet with the oil every night.

File away the offender. Soak your feet in warm water, then use a pumice stone to remove the hardened skin. Don't try to file away the entire corn in one sitting; you'll only irritate the skin. Instead, work at the corn a little bit each night until it's gone.

Foot Odor

Like other body parts, your feet perspire. But the perspiration itself doesn't make your feet smell. Rather, moisture that gets trapped in your shoes enables bacteria to grow, which create the offending odor. Here's what to do.

Roll away the odor. For a quick fix, apply your underarm deodorant to the bottom of your feet. It will fight bacterial odor, although it won't control wetness.

Massage with essential oils. Lavender and tea tree oils are potent antimicrobials, so they'll kill the bacteria that are causing foot odor. The oils smell good too. You can buy them in health food stores and bath-and-beauty shops. Apply one of these oils (dilute 15 drops in a carrier oil) at bedtime, rubbing enough into your feet to coat the skin. Slip on socks to protect your sheets. Repeat the treatment for at least 4 consecutive nights.

Drown the stench. Soak your feet in one of the following solutions for 15 to 20 minutes once or twice a day.

- Epsom salts. Add ½ cup of Epsom salts to 1 quart of warm water.
- Tea. Steep a few regular black tea bags in hot water, then add some cool water so that the tea is lukewarm. Black tea has tannins, which help absorb moisture.
- Vinegar. Add ½ cup white vinegar to 1 quart of warm water.

Pamper your footwear. The insides of shoes are dark and damp, an environment in which bacteria thrive. To discourage microbes from making themselves at home in your footwear, follow this advice.

- Alternate your shoes on a daily basis.
- Don't keep your shoes in a closed, dark place like a locker.
- If you exercise daily, alternate two pairs of athletic shoes.

Hammertoes

The name is apropos because hammertoes are caused by beating up our feet by—what else?—wearing tight, pointed-toe shoes.

The shape of the shoe's toebox forces the sides of the foot (the big toe and/or the pinkie toe) to turn inward, crowding the other toes. Sometimes a toe can get squeezed so much that it curls into an arched position. That's a hammertoe.

If you have a hammertoe, surgery can straighten it. But that should be a last resort. Before you do anything so drastic, try these strategies.

Cruel Shoes

In China, where petite feet were once considered beautiful, young girls' feet were bound so that they would remain only a few inches long. Though such a custom is now considered barbaric, some podiatrists would argue that modern women practice their own version of foot binding, thanks to their penchant for too-tight, too-pointed, high-heeled shoes.

"Many women prefer high heels because they think heels look more appropriate with professional clothes," says Pamela Colman, D.P.M., director of health affairs at the American Podiatric Medical Association. "But the majority of these shoes fit so poorly that, over the course of a lifetime, they slowly deform the feet."

When you wear shoes with heels higher than 2 inches, all of your body weight shifts forward onto the balls of your feet and your toes. The constant pressure, especially on your toes, can lead to an array of foot problems, including blisters, calluses, and corns. Also, high heels often have pointed toeboxes. Over time, your toes assume the triangular shape of the toebox, setting the stage for hammertoes, neuromas, and bunions.

Your feet will fare much better if you choose flat and low-heeled shoes with a generous toebox area. Shoes like this distribute your body weight evenly between the balls of your feet and your heels. Your toes are free to help you keep your balance, uninhibited by pain, irritation, or swelling.

Use your marbles. Pick up 20 marbles with your toes three times a day. This exercise strengthens the tendons in your feet, so the hammertoe stays flexible.

Lend some support. A device called a crest pad can keep a hammertoe from curling under. The pad—actually a tapered foam cushion—is placed under the toes and attached to the top of the foot. You can buy crest pads in medical supply stores.

Find accommodating footwear. Make sure that your shoe has a toebox that is high enough and wide enough to allow enough room for your hammertoe.

Neuromas

If walking a certain way causes a quick, sharp shot of pain that could send you through the roof, chances are that you have a neuroma. A neuroma is an enlarged nerve that has a tendency to get in the way of the tiny bones on the ball of your foot (usually around your fourth toe). Pain lets you know when it happens.

If the pain is unbearable, your doctor may recommend cortisone injections, padding, or even surgery. Fortunately, most neuromas can be managed with sensible self-care. Here's what to do.

Treat your feet. When the pain of a neuroma has your feet in a bind, give them a rest and try elevating them. Also, walk barefoot around the house as much as possible.

Provide padding. A ball-of-the-foot support pad placed in your shoe will reduce pressure on the affected nerve. You can buy the pads in drugstores.

Size up your shoes. Wearing a shoe with a low heel (no more than 2 inches) and a wide enough and high enough toebox will alleviate the pressure on your toes. And that will keep your neuroma from hurting.

Repairing an Ingrown Nail

Toenails are made to be as tough as . . . well, nails. So when a toenail happens to dig into the delicate flesh of a tender tootsie, the pain can be pretty intense.

An ingrown toenail usually occurs for one of two reasons. You may have trimmed your nail in such a way that it started growing into the surrounding skin. Or you may have worn a pair of too-tight shoes that squeezed your toes together, pushing nail into skin.

If you have an ingrown toenail, you should start treating it as soon as possible to prevent it from becoming infected. Here's what doctors suggest you do.

1. Add 1 to 2 tablespoons of salt to 1 quart of lukewarm water. Soak your feet for 15 to 20 minutes. This softens the nail and the skin around it. It also helps fight infection.

Sore Feet

The average woman puts approximately 500 pounds of pressure on her feet just by walking. Multiply that by about 10,000 steps a day, and the stage is set for sore feet.

Put icing on the ache. To reduce inflammation, apply ice to your feet for 15 to 20 minutes once or twice a day. Wrap the ice in a towel so that it doesn't touch your skin. Continue the treatment for 2 to 3 consecutive days.

Play toe tennis. Stand with your foot on a tennis ball. Working from the center of your heel, move the ball down either side of your heel toward the ball of your foot. Massaging your foot in this way relaxes the muscles and tissues

2. With a rounded toothpick, carefully lift the edge of the ingrown toenail as much as you can tolerate. Then slide a small piece of gauze or cotton under the nail where it's digging into your skin. This will encourage the nail to grow out and over the gauze or cotton. If you are unable to do this step, see your doctor.
3. Change the gauze or cotton every day until your toe heals.

While your toe is on the mend, keep it uncovered as much as possible. Take off your shoes and socks or stockings when you're at home, and wear sandals when you can. Also, don't bandage your toe. If you notice any redness, pus, or swelling or if the toe feels more tender after a couple of days, see your doctor.

in the arch of your foot and spreads the metatarsals, the bones in the ball of your foot.

Roll a can for relief. To soothe an aching arch, roll your bare foot over a can of frozen juice concentrate for 5 to 10 minutes. Wrap the can in a towel so that it doesn't touch your skin. The massage helps loosen tense tissues, while the cold helps reduce inflammation.

Stretch out tension. If you have pain between your toes or in the ball of your foot, try this exercise. Lace your fingers between your toes and stretch your toes apart very gently. This exercise helps keep your toes flexible and gives the connective tissue in your feet a good stretch.

Plenty of Reasons to Smile

Proper self-care can prevent most, if not all, tooth and gum problems. Poor dental hygiene can lead to trouble, starting with gingivitis and ending with periodontitis, serious gum deterioration that can result in tooth loss if it is not treated in time. To nip tooth problems in the bud, here's what to do.

Gingivitis

Gingivitis is a form of gum disease caused when dental plaque (a gluelike film of bacteria, food, and saliva) invades the warm and inviting crevasses at and below the gum line. There it hardens into tartar (sometimes called calculus), triggering inflammation and infection.

Left untreated, gingivitis can lead to periodontitis, a condition characterized by severely receding gums and, ultimately, destruction of the jawbone, which anchors your teeth in place. But gingivitis doesn't have to get nearly that far. Combine the following strategies with regular brushing and flossing to combat gingivitis and keep your gums in the pink. If your gums bleed each time you brush, make an appointment to see your dentist.

Make your own herbal toothpaste. Mix 1 tablespoon of the herb goldenseal in dried form with enough water to form a paste. Then brush your teeth with it as you normally would. Goldenseal, which is available in health food stores, can help heal inflamed, diseased gums. (If you are allergic to plants in the daisy family, goldenseal may cause an allergic reaction.)

Brush with baking soda. Mix baking soda with enough hydrogen peroxide to form a paste. With your toothbrush, gently rub the mixture onto your gums. Leave it on for a few minutes, then rinse.

Sip a soothing tea. Add 2 tablespoons of the dried herb anise and 2 tablespoons of dried sage (both sold in health food stores) to 1 cup of freshly boiled water. Allow the herbs to steep for 10 minutes, then strain the tea and drink up. Repeat as needed to relieve sore gums.

Be generous with garlic. Garlic is nature's antibiotic. It helps to fight plaque-forming bacteria, which means that they are less likely to set up shop in your mouth. You can increase your intake of fresh garlic simply by adding it to most of your meals. Worried about garlic breath? Take supplements instead—250 milligrams a day.

Take your Q. Coenzyme Q_{10} is a natural compound that may help treat gingivitis and can promote healthy gum tissue by increasing the flow of oxygen to cells. You will find coenzyme Q_{10} supplements in health food stores.

Sing for high C. Vitamin C can help gum tissue resist the bacterial onslaught that leads to gingivitis. Take 500 milligrams three times a day.

Note: Some people develop diarrhea when taking high doses of vitamin C. If this happens, cut back your dosage to a tolerable level.

Tooth Discoloration

Beginning in their late thirties, many people notice that their once pearly whites are taking on a different hue. Teeth naturally lose some of their outermost layer—the enamel—over the years. And because the material beneath the enamel is darker, your bright smile begins to fade.

Unless you have a calcium deficiency, which will require a doctor's intervention, tooth discoloration is essentially a cosmetic problem. The following tips discourage stains and spiff up your smile.

Whiten wisely. As a natural alternative to home bleaching kits, which can irritate gums, look in your health food store for a product called Peelu. It's a whitener made from tree root extract and sold as a toothpaste and a powder.

Raging Hormones, Bleeding Gums?

Menstruation, pregnancy, menopause, and birth control pills all cause hormonal changes that reduce the ability of a woman's gum tissues to fight the bacteria that cause gingivitis.

Bleeding gums can also signal that a woman's physical and emotional health is out of balance, says Andrea Brockman, D.D.S., board member of the Holistic Dental Association in practice at the Valley Green Center for Holistic Dentistry in Philadelphia. Chronic stress, poor diet, and inadequate sleep can weaken the immune system, allowing gum-damaging bacteria to thrive.

To avoid bleeding gums, you should cut back on red meat, sugar, processed foods, caffeine, and alcohol, says Dr. Brockman. "They can make saliva extremely acidic,

Chew gum as a chaser. After drinking coffee or tea, chew a stick of sugarless gum. This stimulates the production of saliva to help wash away the beverage's residues before they stain.

Sip water to stop stains. Out of gum? Then take a swig of water and swish it around your mouth. Water is enough to clean your teeth and prevent stains from building up.

Tooth Grinding

Most folks who grind their teeth don't even know they do it until someone else tells them about it. That's because tooth grinding (also called bruxism) often occurs during sleep.

Tooth grinding can lead to a variety of problems, including headaches, jaw pain, tooth sensitivity, and

and bacteria thrive in an acidic environment." Avoid smoking, and eat more fish, whole grains, and raw fruits and vegetables.

For already sore gums, turn to tea tree, lavender, eucalyptus, or peppermint essential oil to inhibit the growth of bacteria and speed away infection, advises Dr. Brockman. If you use a pulsating irrigation device such as a Water Pik or Hydro Floss, add up to five drops of one of these oils to about ⅔ cup of distilled water and place in the reservoir. "The oils will penetrate and stay in the gingival tissues," says Dr. Brockman.

As an alternative, mix up to five drops of one of the oils with a few ounces of distilled water and swish it around in your mouth two or three times a day. (Essential oils can be toxic if swallowed, so don't use this on children.)

temporomandibular disorder, in which the hinges of the jaw malfunction. If you routinely have tooth or face pain when you wake up, see a dentist.

Fortunately, you can do things while you're awake to soothe a painful jaw and break the tooth-grinding habit. Here's what dentists recommend.

Get immediate relief with heat. Soak a towel in warm water, wring it out, and wrap it around a hot-water bottle. Apply this compress to your face for 15 to 20 minutes, frequently checking your skin to make sure that it's not getting burned.

Sip herbal tea before snoozing. Considering a nightcap to help you relax? Some research suggests that drinking alcohol before going to bed can worsen tooth grinding. Have a cup of herbal tea instead.

Follow the dots. Go to your nearest office supply store and buy a sheet or two of orange dot stickers. Paste them everywhere: on your mirror, your dashboard, and your refrigerator door. Every time you see one, take it as your cue to separate your teeth. This simple trick discourages tooth grinding.

Tooth Sensitivity

Its lightning bolt of pain can turn a sweet experience, like sipping an ice-cold glass of lemonade, sour real fast.

If you have a sensitive tooth, you may decide to deal with it by avoiding whatever triggers your pain. That's fine for a temporary fix, but you really need to have the tooth checked out by your dentist to determine what's wrong. In the meantime, these self-care measures can minimize your discomfort.

Pass the jelly. Petroleum jelly doesn't feel or taste very good inside your mouth, but it quiets a sensitive tooth on a short-term basis. Simply apply petroleum jelly to the tooth.

Extend an olive branch. If tooth sensitivity results from an abrasion or erosion along the gum line, olive oil can help. Warm the oil by pouring a small amount into a saucepan and slightly heating it. Dampen a cotton swab in the oil, then wave the swab in the air briefly to cool it off. Dry the affected tooth with a tissue or cotton ball and then dab the warm oil on your gum line a couple of times. Repeat as needed. (One treatment may last for months.)

Take a hard look at soft drinks. If you're drinking enough colas and root beers to float an armada, cut back. The darker sodas have high levels of phosphoric acid, which pulls calcium out of your body—and your teeth—like crazy.

Switch to a softer brush. A tooth can become sensitive because of overly aggressive brushing, especially with a brush that has hard bristles. This combination can push back the gum and expose the root surface. Use a toothbrush with softer bristles, and adopt a gentler brushing technique.

Chapped Lips

For all the wear and tear that they endure, lips are remarkably unprotected. They lack the natural oils that keep the rest of your skin supple. They also lack melanin, the pigment that provides some protection against sun damage. And exposure to blazing sun, strong winds, or moisture-sapping indoor heat causes plenty of chapping.

A few days of TLC—tender lip care—is all you should need to restore the wetness to your whistle. Here's what to do. (If you have severely cracked lips, see your doctor. You may need a prescription preparation.)

Smear on the old standby. For chapped lips, nothing works better than petroleum jelly.

Brushing and Flossing: Do It Right

Thoroughly brushing your teeth takes at least 3 minutes—not the 51 seconds that most women allow. Brushing *and* flossing prevent the formation of plaque, a sticky film that coats teeth and eventually causes cavities and gingivitis (swollen, bleeding gums).

To brush properly, follow these three steps, then finish by brushing the surface of your tongue, which can harbor bacteria and contribute to bad breath.

1. Position the brush at a 45-degree angle to your gum line. Use short back-and-forth strokes to clean the outside of your teeth and then the inside.
2. Brush the chewing surfaces of your teeth.
3. Clean the inside of your front teeth by holding the brush perpendicular to your jaw. Move the brush from the gum toward the biting edge—up on your lower teeth, down on your upper teeth.

Ideally, your teeth should be brushed five times a day: in the morning, at bedtime, and after each meal. At least one of those sessions should be followed by flossing. Be sure to pick the right floss for you. If you have rough fill-

Thumb your nose at dryness. If you have oily skin and you're outdoors with no lip balm handy, run your finger along the side of your nose to pick up some skin oil. Wipe the oil on your lips for short-term relief.

Fight yeast with yogurt. If the corners of your mouth appear red and cracked, you may have an overgrowth of yeast (a fungus), caused perhaps by antibiotics or stress. Go to the supermarket and pick up some yogurt containing live active cultures (check the label). Swish the

ings or if your teeth are close together, waxed floss works best. Unwaxed floss is thinner than waxed, but it also frays more readily. If your teeth are widely spaced or if you have a hard time flossing, dental tape is a good choice.

To practice proper flossing, follow these five steps.

1. Tear off a strand of floss about 18 inches long. Wrap the ends around the middle fingers of both hands until just 6 to 8 inches of floss is exposed.
2. Pinch the floss between the thumb and index finger of one hand. With the index finger of your other hand, guide about 1 inch of floss between your teeth.
3. Use a back-and-forth motion as you gently slide the floss up and down between your teeth.
4. Curve the floss around the base of each tooth. Gently move the floss back and forth beneath the gum line.
5. To remove the floss, use the same back-and-forth motion to bring it up and away from your teeth. Never snap or force the floss, or you might bruise delicate gum tissue.

yogurt around in your mouth several times a day. The live active cultures include *Lactobacillus acidophilus*, beneficial bacteria that control yeast.

Cover up your kisser. Always apply a lip balm with a sun protection factor (SPF) of 15 or higher before heading outside.

Lick your problem, not your lips. Licking your lips to moisturize them is only natural. Unfortunately, air evaporates the moisture, leaving your lips even drier than before.

Cold Sores

Nothing can ruin a beautiful smile like a nasty-looking cold sore. And if you get one once, you're likely to get them again and again.

You can credit their persistence to herpes simplex type 1, the virus that causes cold sores. Ninety percent of the people who carry the virus picked it up during childhood. It lurks in your system forever, lying dormant among the nerve ganglia beneath your skin's surface, just waiting for something to activate it.

For many people, that something is usually stress. When you're under stress, your resistance to disease drops. The virus seizes the opportunity to instigate an outbreak.

A cold sore usually sticks around for 1 to 2 weeks. You can use these natural remedies to minimize any discomfort and shorten the duration of an outbreak.

Give it the cold shoulder. The minute you feel a cold sore coming on, wrap an ice cube in a handkerchief and hold it directly on the sore for about 5 minutes. Repeat every 2 to 3 hours. No virus, including herpes simplex type 1, can survive in a cold environment.

Try a little tenderizer. Mix meat tenderizer with a few drops of water to make a paste. Apply the paste to the cold sore and hold it in place with a dry washcloth for 5 to 10 minutes. Repeat every 2 to 3 hours for the first day of an outbreak, then cut back the treatments to three times a day. Continue until the sore heals.

Line up lysine. Before the advent of the prescription drug acyclovir (Zovirax) for cold sores, people swore by the preventive and healing properties of lysine. This amino acid counteracts arginine, a substance in various foods that seems to trigger cold sores in some people. Lysine tablets are available in drugstores and health food stores.

Shrink the sore with zinc. An essential trace mineral, zinc is essential for proper wound healing—especially cell production—and helps get rid of cold sores more quickly. During an outbreak, take 30 milligrams of zinc a day with food or water. Once the sore heals, cut back to 15 milligrams a day.

Note: If you're taking more than 20 milligrams daily, it's a good idea to inform your doctor.

Dab on some sun protection. If you have had a cold sore in the past, wearing lip balm with an SPF of 30 at all times can help prevent another outbreak. You can find lip balms with high SPFs in sporting goods stores and drugstores. (During an outbreak, use a cotton swab to apply the balm to your lips and the outside border of the cold sore. That way, you won't transfer the virus to the balm stick.)

Leave it alone. If you have a cold sore, don't pull it, stretch it, or otherwise touch it. You could get very painful cold sores on your hand, especially if the fluid from the blister gets under a hangnail.

Relief for Sore Eyes

Of all six senses, we rely on vision the most. In fact, a full 80 percent of the information that we gather from the world around us passes through our eyes.

With that kind of activity, our eyes are entitled to get a little tired and sore from time to time. But these days, eye problems seem more prevalent than ever. That's because we're devoting more time to what optometrists call near-point tasks—things such as gazing at computer and TV screens and reading the tiny type in stock reports and on food labels. Unfortunately, human eyes weren't designed for this kind of up-close work.

"Most common eye conditions—including bloodshot eyes and eyestrain—can have a functional cause, meaning that they occur because of the way we use our eyes," explains Anne Barber, O.D., director of program services for the Optometric Extension Program Foundation, an organization based in Santa Ana, California, that promotes vision education. "They're characteristic of a visual system that isn't functioning as efficiently as it should."

Regular exams are your best eye insurance because

they'll catch any vision changes—as well as serious conditions such as cataracts, glaucoma, and macular degeneration—early on. Dr. Barber suggests that you see an optometrist or ophthalmologist every 2 years until you reach age 55, then every year thereafter. "If we catch a problem early on and start treating it right away, we stand a better chance of saving vision. So be sure your vision care provider does a full series of near-point vision tests and provides vision therapy to take care of functional problems or refers you to an office that does," she says.

For more run-of-the-mill eye conditions, proper self-care is usually sufficient. Eye doctors share these favorite natural remedies for keeping the eyes and eye area healthy.

Bloodshot Eyes

As eye problems go, bloodshot eyes are easy to self-diagnose. You just have to look in the mirror. To bring those blood vessels down to size and get rid of the redness, follow this advice.

Clear your eyes with cold. Wrap ice cubes in a clean washcloth and lay the compress over your eyes for 30 minutes.

Buy tears in a bottle. Artificial tears ease the sting of bloodshot eyes and clear up the irritation that made you see red in the first place. You'll find these products in drugstores. (If you wear contacts, rewetting drops work just as well.)

Dispense with the medicated eyedrops. Funny thing about over-the-counter medicated eyedrops such as Visine or Murine: The more you use them, the more you need them. It's a condition that doctors call rebound hyperemia. Reserve medicated eyedrops for occasional use.

Eyedrops Made Easy

Here's the no-fuss, no-drip way to self-administer eyedrops, from Anne Sumers, M.D., an ophthalmologist in Ridgewood, New Jersey, and spokesperson for the American Academy of Ophthalmology.

Tilt your head back or lie down on the couch. Pull your lower lid away from your eye so that it forms a little pocket. Then squeeze the eyedrop into the pocket. Do not let the dropper touch your eye or eyelid. Bacteria can contaminate the eyedropper if it touches you. Contact with the dropper can also scratch your cornea.

Do the second eye immediately after the first. Then close your eyes for a minute or two and press your index fingers next to the corners of your eyes where they meet your nose. This closes the drainage duct between your eye and nose so the drops stay where they belong. Keeping your eyes open or blinking sends the drops into the duct. If that happens, your eye won't benefit from the drops at all. (And if you're using a type of prescription drops called a beta-blocker and it goes down into that duct, you could experience a slow or irregular heartbeat, notes Dr. Sumers.)

Before opening your eyes, wipe away any lingering moisture from your closed lids. Finally, if you don't think the drop got into your eye, do it again. You can't overdose on eyedrops, says Dr. Sumers.

Crow's-Feet

The first signs of crow's-feet usually appear when we reach our late twenties. At that point, the tiny lines are visible only when we squint. They gradually deepen over the years and become prominent once we reach our forties.

The sooner you take steps to prevent crow's-feet, the younger the skin around your eyes will appear. But even if you already have lines, you can minimize their appearance.

Fade lines with AHAs. Alpha hydroxy acids (AHAs)—natural acids derived from foods such as fruits, sugarcane, and sour milk—diminish crow's-feet by sloughing off old skin cells and exposing younger cells underneath. AHAs also plump the skin and restore its ability to retain moisture. Look for an eye cream containing 5 percent AHAs. (Be careful to avoid your eyelids when applying.)

Switch from alpha to beta. If you have sensitive skin, use a product containing beta hydroxy acids. They reduce fine lines and wrinkles just as well as AHAs but with less irritation.

Invest in cool shades. Always wear wraparound sunglasses in bright or hazy outdoor light. Sunglasses may help prevent crow's-feet by stopping you from squinting.

Stop rubbing your eyes. The skin around your eyes can stretch and wrinkle in response to repeated rubbing.

Dark Circles

Contrary to popular belief, heredity—not lack of sleep—typically paints that bluish black or brownish tinge on the skin. While fatigue doesn't cause dark circles, it can certainly make them more pronounced. So can excessive sun exposure, as the sun's rays break down collagen and elastin. Allergies, illness, menstruation, and even pregnancy can also aggravate existing dark circles.

Medically speaking, dark circles under the eyes are harmless. Still, if you have them, you probably wish they were a little less noticeable. They can be, if you follow this advice.

Count on chamomile. Chamomile helps minimize dark circles by constricting the blood vessels, including those under the eyes. Place a steeped, chilled chamomile tea bag under each closed eye for 10 to 20 minutes in the morning while you're waiting for the coffee to brew.

Note: Some pollen-sensitive people may be allergic to chamomile tea. Discontinue use if you experience any negative reaction.

Let witch hazel do the work. As an alternative to chamomile, soak cotton balls in witch hazel and lay them on the skin under your closed eyes for 20 minutes.

Keep them hidden. To cover dark circles, use a yellow-based stick concealer. Yellow neutralizes pink, red, and purple hues in the skin.

Eye Irritations

Unless you wear protective goggles 24 hours a day, you're eventually going to get something in your eye. It could be a speck of dust, grit, or makeup. The longer it stays put, the redder, scratchier, and more swollen your eye will become.

Foreign objects aren't the only things that irritate eyes. Smoke, pollen, and chlorine (in swimming pools) do the job just as well. If you have removed an irritant yet you have discharge coming from your eye, or other abnormal symptoms, see your ophthalmologist. Irritation can also arise from a bacterial or viral infection.

Whatever its cause, eye irritation can usually be treated at home with simple self-care techniques. Here's what to do.

Flip your lid. If something is in your eye, you can use your eyelids to gently push the particle down and out. Grasp the eyelashes of your upper lid between your fingers, then pull the upper lid over the lower lid. This allows the lower lashes to brush the speck off the inside of your upper lid. If the particle moves to the corner of your eye, remove it with the corner of a moist tissue.

Let the water flow. Ordinary tap water can flush a foreign object from your eye. Go to the sink, lean down close to the faucet, and splash water into your eye.

Be bold with cold. For irritation caused by an allergy, lay a washcloth soaked in fresh cold water over your eyes for 5 to 10 minutes.

Make a shampoo solution. Eye irritation sometimes results from blepharitis, a condition in which the eyelid margin (the thin edge of skin between your eyeball and eyelashes) becomes swollen from excess oil production. To treat blepharitis, add two or three drops of no-tears baby shampoo to ⅓ cup of water, dip a cotton swab into the solution, and run the swab along the bottom eyelid margin while your eye is open. Then close your eye and run the swab over the top eyelid margin where the lid meets the eyelashes. Use this remedy once or twice a day.

Pinkeye

Feel as though a mosquito is permanently lodged underneath your eyelid? Are the whites of your eyes so irritated that they've turned pink or bloodshot red? Odds are that you have pinkeye.

Typically, pinkeye results from an allergy to pollen, pet dander, or certain chemicals or from a bacterial or viral infection. In fact, the same viruses that cause the common cold can also cause pinkeye. And like the common cold, infectious pinkeye is extremely contagious and easily spread by hand-to-eye contact.

Bacterial pinkeye is the most serious type, and unless it's treated with prescription medication, it can lead to loss of vision.

Seeing a doctor at the first sign of pinkeye is important. She can decide whether you require a prescription or you can manage the condition with self-care alone. Then use these strategies to help relieve the immediate symptoms and prevent the spread of germs.

Remove your contacts. If you wear contacts, take them out at the first sign of redness and irritation. Otherwise, they'll only worsen your discomfort, and if you have infectious pinkeye, they'll trap the germs in your eyes.

Run hot and cold. Alternating hot and cold compresses stimulates circulation and draws infection-fighting white blood cells to your eyes. Soak a clean washcloth in very warm water, wring it out, and hold it against your eyes for a minute. Then soak the cloth in cold water, wring it out, and hold it against your eyes for a minute. Repeat this process two or three times.

Check out chickweed. The herb chickweed helps fight infection, yet it's mild enough to use on your eyes. Brew a pot of chickweed tea and let it cool until it is comfortable to the touch. Then dip a clean cloth into the tea and hold the cloth against the affected eye while it's closed. Continue rewetting and reapplying the cloth for up to an hour.

Get goldenseal. If you have bacterial pinkeye, an eye bath of goldenseal tea can soothe your eyes and fight the infection. To make the eye bath, add 1 teaspoon of dried goldenseal to 1 cup of freshly boiled water. Steep for 10 minutes, then strain the mixture and allow the liquid to cool. Use an eyedropper to squirt two drops of the liquid into the affected eye.

Leave your eyes *au naturel*. Avoid wearing eye makeup while you have infectious pinkeye. Replace your mascara and liner. If your mascara wand or liner becomes contaminated, you'll just keep transferring the virus or bacteria from one eye to the other.

Sties

Each of your eyelids contains eyelash follicles. Sometimes one of these follicles becomes infected, perhaps because it's clogged with dandrufflike scales or you have used a germ-laden mascara brush. Eventually, a painful red lump with a white head of pus sprouts at the base of the eyelash. This is what's known as a sty.

If you have a persistent or recurrent sty, see your doctor. It could be a sign of diabetes or a cyst. Also see a doctor if your sty doesn't get better or gets worse after 2 days.

As with a pimple on your face, a sty should never be popped. It may rupture beneath the surface of the skin, aggravating the inflammation. Instead, heed this advice.

Hold a hot potato. Wrap a warm, damp washcloth around a hot baked potato (the cloth will retain the heat longer). Then hold the cloth against the affected, closed eye for 5 minutes. Repeat four times every day for 2 weeks. This will gently coax the sty to break open and heal.

Give your eyes a break. Stop wearing eye makeup until the sty heals. This means *all* eye makeup—mascara, eyeliner, and shadow. Otherwise, you may end up with several sties.

Tired Eyes

Tired eyes, while uncomfortable, are seldom cause for alarm. Still, if your discomfort persists, you should see an ophthalmologist. You may need eyeglasses for when you do close work.

To perk up tired eyes, try these tips.

Look around. The moment your eyes begin to bother you, look up from your work and into the distance. This lets your eye muscles relax.

Put your palms to work. Rub your hands together to warm them up a bit. Then gently position your palms over your closed eyes. Hold for 5 minutes, breathing easily while you do. This should rest and rejuvenate your eyes quite nicely.

FOLK REMEDY: DOES IT WORK?

Cucumber Slices for Puffy Eyes

"Puffy eyes are induced by things like crying, menstruation, and other factors that may cause the body to retain fluid," says Mary Ruth Buchness, M.D., chief of dermatology at St. Vincent's Hospital and Medical Center in New York City. Cucumbers won't take the fluid away, and they may even make your eyes feel worse. They contain a substance that in some women can cause an immediate reaction in the form of hives.

Recommendation: Forget It

Squeeze out fatigue. Take a deep breath while raising your shoulders and squeezing your eyes and fists as tightly closed as you can. Then exhale and relax all of the muscles at once. By tightening and releasing the voluntary muscles in your shoulders and fists, you can trick the involuntary muscles in your eyes into releasing as well.

Under-Eye Bags

Baggy eyes develop with age. As you grow older, the muscles under your eyes weaken, and the skin becomes less elastic. Fat tissue pushes through and around the muscles, giving the skin a swollen appearance. Once bags develop, you can't do much about them other than concealing them with makeup or having cosmetic surgery.

Puffy eyes, on the other hand, are temporary. They occur when something prompts your body to collect and retain fluid under the eyes. That something could be almost anything, including crying, lack of sleep, allergies, menstruation, or eating salty foods. If you awaken and find one eye swollen three times greater than the other, call your physician. This could be a sign of hives or an allergic reaction to an insect bite. In addition, visit your doctor if your eyes don't close all the way (it could indicate thyroid disease).

As with baggy eyes, you can use makeup to mask puffy eyes. But to get rid of the puffiness for good, try these strategies.

Spoon on relief. One of the fastest, easiest, and cheapest ways to reduce puffiness around your eyes is with a glass of ice water and four metal serving spoons. Chill the spoons in the ice water, then place one spoon over each eye. When the spoons become warm, switch them with the others chilling in the glass of water.

Make tea bag compresses. Tea contains tannins, natural astringents that pull skin taut and reduce puffiness. Wrap two steeped, cooled tea bags in tissue (so they won't stain your skin), then lay the bags over your closed eyes for 2 to 5 minutes.

Dry out with dandelion. A natural diuretic, the dandelion herb helps your body eliminate excess fluid. Three times a day, drink a cup of dandelion leaf tea or take ½ teaspoon of dandelion leaf tincture. You can buy herbal tinctures, dried herbs, or teas in health food stores.

Note: Women who are taking diuretics, such as for high blood pressure, should not drink dandelion tea. And if you have gallbladder disease, do not use it without your doctor's okay.

Super Nail Solutions

The computer revolution has had at least one unexpected and as yet unexplained health benefit for women. All that tap-tap-tapping on computer keyboards appears to make fingernails grow faster and stronger.

Even if you're not computer-crazed, any activity that has you striking your nails against a hard surface—from playing the piano to drumming your fingers—can stimulate growth, according to Diana Bihova, M.D., a dermatologist in New York City and author of *Beauty from the Inside Out*. So can menstruation and pregnancy. "Weather is a factor, too," she says. "We don't know exactly why, but fingernails grow faster in summer."

Hard As Nails

Of course, moving to warmer climes isn't the most practical way to get longer, stronger nails. Thankfully, you have more sensible options. The following strategies can keep your nails looking their best.

Trim after you bathe. Cutting your nails while they're dry leaves them vulnerable to damage. Instead, plan your manicure for after your bath or shower, when your nails are soft.

Avoid cutting corners. When trimming your nails, leave them square at the corners. This maximizes nail strength.

File away flaws. Keep an emery board in your purse or desk drawer. At the first sign of a nick or chip, use the board to smooth out the unevenness and prevent further damage. Always file in the same direction.

Slather on moisturizer. Apply moisturizer to your hands every time you wash them. Take a moment to massage the lotion into your skin and nails.

Be prudent with polish remover. Frequent use of nail polish remover can dry out your nails. So use remover sparingly, preferably no more than once a week. Look for an acetone-free product, which is less drying. Apply a small amount to a cotton ball, press it against your nail for about 2 seconds, and then gently rub off the polish.

Protect your mitts. Whenever you wash dishes or use household cleaners, wear protective latex gloves with separate thin cotton gloves underneath. The cotton gloves help absorb perspiration. That's important because sweat makes hands soggy, further weakening nails.

Brittle Nails

It's doubtful that anyone will go through life without getting brittle nails. Some of us are born with them. Others get them after years of submerging their hands in water or harsh household detergents. Growing older takes a toll, too: Almost everyone's nails become thinner with age.

So what can you do to restore moisture to your nails and keep them healthy and strong? For starters, try these tips.

A Manicure for Healthy Nails

Here's the best way to buff and shine your nails to perfect health, according to Ida Orengo, M.D., associate professor of dermatology at Baylor College of Medicine in Houston.

- First, place your hands in a small dish of warm water mixed with mild detergent for 5 minutes to remove dirt and bacteria. "This gets your nails fresh and clean and avoids the possibility of pushing any bacteria under your cuticles," says Dr. Orengo. Dry your hands gently with a soft, clean towel.
- While your nails are still soft, gently cut or clip them to about ¼ inch in length. Anything longer can break, split, and chip more easily.
- With an orange stick wrapped in cotton gauze, gently push back your cuticles. Cuticles should never be cut, says Dr. Orengo, because they protect your nails against bacterial and fungal infections.
- File your nails with an emery board while they're soft and pliable. File in one direction, from side to center, until they are squared off at the top. Filing in a back-and-forth motion can weaken nails, as can filing them to a point.
- Rub your nails liberally with a nail moisturizing lotion to hydrate them and prevent drying and cracking. Wait 2 or 3 minutes for the moisturizer to soak into your nails, then wipe off the excess.
- Before applying color, brush on a clear precoat polish to prevent your nails from turning yellow.

Offer 'em olive oil. Immerse your fingertips in ½ cup of warmed olive oil and soak for 15 to 30 minutes.

Break open the bath beads. As an alternative to olive oil, break open three or four bath-oil capsules, and empty their contents into ½ cup of warm water. Soak your fingertips in the diluted bath oil for 5 minutes.

Make bedtime a formal affair. Before going to bed, coat your nails and hands with a thick layer of petroleum jelly. Then slip on a pair of white cotton gloves to protect your hands overnight. You'll love the way this treatment makes your nails look.

Go for a quick fix. To salvage a split or broken nail, apply a very small amount of nail glue to the tear. Reinforce the tear by covering it with a small piece of tissue from a tea bag. Let the glue dry completely, then use a fine buffer to even out the nail surface. (Be sure to leave the tissue in place.) Finally, apply a top coat over the tissue.

Hangnails

A hangnail forms when a small piece of skin tears away from your finger right by the nail bed. Even though it's tiny, it can be quite painful and even bleed.

If you get a hangnail, don't pick at it or try to bite it off. It can actually become infected. To remove a hangnail the right way, use this three-step technique.

Start by softening. Never cut off a hangnail while it's dry. Instead, soften it by soaking it in a mixture of warm water and olive oil.

Clip it cleanly. Use nail scissors or nail clippers to remove the hangnail. Cut it as short as you can without damaging the skin around it.

Apply the finishing touches. After clipping the hangnail, massage the skin around your nail with moisturizer, cover it with an adhesive bandage, and leave it alone.

Sore Cuticles

That tiny rim of near-transparent tissue at the base of each nail is there for a reason. It serves as a barrier, protecting the nail against infection.

To repair damaged cuticles and keep them problem-free, add these steps to your nail-care routine.

First, soak them. Before you do anything to your cuticles, soften them in warm, sudsy water for several minutes. This prevents drying and cracking.

Then give them a gentle push. Wrap the tip of an orange stick in cotton gauze. Then use the stick to gently push back each cuticle.

Finish with petroleum jelly. After pushing back your cuticles, massage them with a thin layer of petroleum jelly to seal in moisture.

Part Three

Your Body

Banish the Monthly Blues

If there's anything that a woman can depend on to be undependable, it's her period. It may arrive like clockwork each month, but how it's going to act is anyone's guess. Menstrual symptoms seem to have minds of their own.

To deal with these constant yet ever-changing facts of life, many women turn to old standbys such as ibuprofen and over-the-counter diuretics. While usually good for pain and for water retention, these medications don't treat all the symptoms that bother women—and they can have unwanted side effects.

Healthy lifestyle changes such as eating right and exercising can prevent problems that come with your period. For natural solutions to monthly problems, try the following.

Cramps

For almost half of us, our periods announce their arrival with some kind of pain. It can last for as little as an hour or as long as 3 days. Why?

When hormones called prostaglandins are released during your period, the uterine blood vessels constrict and decrease bloodflow to the area. As a result, the uterine muscle clenches tightly, and you feel it as a cramp.

Many of the world's traditional, natural healing systems treat cramps successfully.

Calm cramps with herbs. Black haw and cramp bark both have a long history of use to relax the muscles of the uterus. If your cramps are mild, make a tea: Add 2 teaspoons of dried black haw or cramp bark per cup of water. Boil for 10 minutes, cool, and strain; drink up to three cups a day.

Severe cramps may require stronger medicine. Try 1 teaspoon of black haw or cramp bark tincture (sometimes labeled as an herbal extract) every half-hour for 2 to 3 hours. It is best not to wait until your pain peaks to start dosing.

If you are routinely plagued with cramps, you should start taking the herbs a few days before you expect your period. Since these herbs, which can be purchased at health food stores, contain an aspirin-like compound, do not use them if you are sensitive to aspirin. Don't take black haw if you have a history of kidney stones.

Heat things up. Lying in a tub of hot water helps relax tense uterine muscles, thereby easing your cramps.

As an alternative, you can make your own heating pad. Dampen a terry-cloth towel in comfortably hot water. Wring it out and test it for temperature before placing it over your crampy lower abdomen. Then relax and let the towel cool naturally.

Relieve pressure with pressure. Press the traditional Chinese acupressure points for relieving menstrual cramps. These points are located at the groin, in the middle of the crease where each of your legs joins your trunk. You can press there with your fingertips, or you can stimulate both points at once by positioning your left fist over the points on your left side and your right fist on the right side. Then, lying on your stomach with your fists in place, use the weight of your body to apply pressure to the areas for at least 2 minutes.

Pour a glass of water. Scientific research shows that increased hydration relieves menstrual cramps. If you have cramps, drink as much water as you can until the cramps go away.

Stretch out. Your lower back and thighs may ache when cramps stimulate nerves that supply these areas. Stretching yoga-style can help.

Sit on the floor with your legs together and stretched in front of you, your arms by your sides with your hands touching the floor. Bend your right leg out to the side and bring your foot next to your left inner thigh.

Inhale. Push into the floor with your hands to lift your chest and lengthen your spine upward; twist your torso to the left so that your breastbone is directly over your extended leg. As you exhale, bend forward from the hips, keeping your back straight. Reach forward and grasp your left foot with both hands (use a belt instead of your hands if necessary). Do not hunch your spine. Stay stretched for 2 to 3 minutes.

Give yourself a rubdown. For quick relief, add five drops each of warming, muscle-relaxing essential oils of wintergreen and lavender to 1 tablespoon of olive or almond oil. Rub it over your abdomen or lower back, then apply a heating pad—for no more than 20 minutes at a time—covered by a thin towel and set on low.

Endometriosis Pain

Normally, the endometrial tissue—the soft, blood-rich lining of a woman's uterus—thickens and is shed each month. But in some women, endometrial tissue migrates outside the uterus and starts to grow on and around other pelvic organs, such as the ovaries, colon, and bladder, or the fallopian tubes.

The renegade tissue may exert pressure on the organs and result in pain. Endometriosis may also lead to painful sex, infertility, or both.

Endometriosis can't be cured, but you can control the pain and possibly the growth of the tissue by natural means. Here's how.

Practice relaxation. By systematically tensing and relaxing individual muscle groups in your body, you can release tension and slow the cycle of pain, stress, and more pain. Close your eyes, take a few deep breaths, and tense the muscles in your face. Hold for a few seconds, then take a deep breath and release. Repeat this for your neck, shoulders, arms, and on down through your body.

Since progressive relaxation needs to be practiced, do it regularly, not just when the pain is bad.

Increase your bioflavonoids. Bioflavonoids seem to reduce excessive bleeding by strengthening capillary walls. These vitamin C–related substances, found in citrus fruits, garlic, onions, and all other vegetables, may also help lower excessively high estrogen levels. So eat your fruit and vegetables and take 1,000 milligrams of bioflavonoids daily as a supplement. Look for bioflavonoids at health food stores.

Cut down on animal fat. Eat less meat, fatty fish and poultry, dairy products, and eggs to reduce your exposure to dioxins, which are chemical residues that may be linked to both the onset and severity of endometriosis.

Buy pads or unbleached tampons. Avoid regular tampons, which owe their pure white appearance to a bleaching process that leaves dioxins behind in the cotton. Switch to sanitary pads or look for 100 percent unbleached, organic cotton tampons.

Is Toxic Shock Syndrome Still a Problem?

Toxic shock syndrome (TSS), a rare but potentially deadly disease associated with tampon use, just isn't as prevalent as it used to be, thanks to new awareness among women who use tampons and perhaps to new standards for tampon absorbency.

While TSS doesn't make the news so often these days, it still affects up to 17 out of every 100,000 menstruating women and girls each year. Experts suspect that this illness is caused by bacteria entering the bloodstream, and it has been linked to the use of high-absorbency tampons. (Tampons seem to create an ideal breeding ground for bacteria.) Some research has shown that 8 out of 10 cases of TSS were among women who used this type of tampon.

You can avoid TSS by choosing the tampon with the minimum absorbency needed to manage your menstrual flow and by changing tampons frequently, says Mary Beth Hasselquist, M.D., clinical assistant professor at the University of Washington in Seattle. Never go more than 8 hours without switching to a fresh one. And don't wear tampons exclusively. Alternating tampons with pads can reduce the risk of TSS. If you experience any warning signs of TSS—sudden fever, vomiting, diarrhea, fainting, dizziness, or a rash that looks like sunburn—remove the tampon immediately and call your doctor.

Heavy Bleeding

An occasional change in your monthly flow is perfectly normal and may be due to a lifestyle change. Have you started a new exercise program? Taken a new job? Moved into a new home?

Age could also be a factor: Your uterus keeps growing until you're around age 35, so there's more uterine lining to bleed. Approaching menopause can also bring unpredictable, heavy periods. You should pay attention to your cycle so you know what's normal for you, and be certain to have an annual examination.

If bleeding or pain seems unusually severe or if you miss a period, see a doctor. If she rules out possible underlying medical causes for heavy bleeding, these suggestions may ease the problem.

Eat iron-rich foods. Inadequate iron intake may cause excessive bleeding. The most efficiently absorbed iron is supplied by foods such as red meat, liver, egg yolks, and fish.

If you're watching your fat intake, a multivitamin/mineral supplement with iron is a sound alternative. Vegetarians can get iron from grains, beans, and dried fruit, but they must also take vitamin C to enhance absorption.

Reach for a raspberry infusion. According to herbal medical lore, a cup a day of raspberry leaf infusion acts as a tonic for the ovaries and uterus. To make it, add about 4 tablespoons of dried raspberry leaves to 1 quart of boiling water, then remove it from the heat and let stand overnight. Strain before drinking.

Mix a bark and valerian cocktail. Heavy bleeding accompanied by nasty cramps responds well to a blend of 3 teaspoons cramp bark tincture and 5 teaspoons valerian tincture. Take between 40 drops and 1 teaspoon of this blend in small amounts of warm water up to three times a day if necessary. Since every woman's cramps are different, the dose that works will be unique as well.

Premenstrual Syndrome

It's not all in your head. You really do want to hang a Do Not Disturb sign around your neck the week before your period. Your cravings for chocolate are utterly overwhelming. And your favorite pants just won't zip shut.

But you've resolved not to give in to premenstrual discomfort. Here's how.

Eat a little—often. Eating five small meals a day, with a good balance of complex carbohydrates and a moderate amount of protein, can ease food cravings and mood swings. Good examples: half a turkey sandwich on whole wheat bread, half a whole wheat bagel spread with low-fat or fat-free cream cheese, a cup of chicken-vegetable soup with whole wheat crackers.

Drink a drop of chasteberry. Take 5 to 15 drops of chasteberry tincture, mixed with a few ounces of water, three times a day. Chasteberry, also called vitex, is commonly prescribed in Europe for PMS.

Maximize your magnesium. Magnesium plays an important part in the treatment of PMS, according to some studies. Taking 300 milligrams of magnesium every day is associated with fewer cramps, less water retention, and an overall improvement in premenstrual symptoms. You'll also find magnesium in nuts, legumes, whole grains, and green vegetables.

Tender Breasts

For most women, breast discomfort waxes and wanes with their menstrual cycles. Right before and during menstruation, higher-than-usual levels of estrogen may cause one or both breasts to swell and become tender. Know your body and what to expect each month. Any unusual increase in pain or discomfort calls for a visit to your doctor.

For tender breasts, here's what to do.

Comfort with a warm compress. Holding a warm compress such as a heated towel or towel-wrapped heating pad against the breast for 10 to 15 minutes can give some relief.

Ice the swelling. For some women, the uncomfortable swelling can be relieved with cold compresses. Wrap ice packs in towels, mold them around your breasts, and keep them there until the packs warm. Repeat as needed.

Keep your glass filled. Drink at least eight 8-ounce glasses of water a day. Paradoxically, the more water you drink, the less likely it is that your breasts will swell before your period.

Get enough fiber. Consume at least 30 grams of fiber a day. Both kinds of fiber—soluble and insoluble—help escort excess estrogen from your body, which prevents the hormone from stimulating breast tissue and causing discomfort.

Reduce your dietary fat. Limit your intake of dietary fat to 15 percent of calories. In one study, women who adhered to this guideline reported significant reductions in breast tenderness, swelling, and lumpiness.

Your Breast Advice

Women need to get into a regular pattern of breast care, says Kathleen Mayzel, M.D., director of the Faulkner Breast Center in Boston. That includes annual visits with your doctor for breast exams, regular mammograms if you're over age 40, and monthly breast self-exams.

But it doesn't end there. You should take the initiative to prevent the thing women fear most: breast cancer. While nothing completely eliminates your risk, you can tilt the odds in your favor.

Preventing Breast Cancer

In Asian countries, breast cancer rates are lower than those in the United States. Research suggests that the Asian diet, which includes less fat and meat and more soy food than ours does, offers significant protection.

Diet has a considerable effect on breast cancer risk. Here are some dietary changes you can make today.

Stay away from alcohol. The more you drink, the higher your risk of breast cancer. Alcohol seems to interfere with your liver's ability to clear excess estrogen from your body. The higher your exposure to estrogen, research finds, the higher your breast cancer risk.

Buy colorful produce. Fruits and vegetables are good sources of cancer-fighting vitamin C and beta-carotene. This is particularly true of the bright orange, yellow, red, and green fruits and vegetables, such as butternut squash, oranges, peaches, sweet red peppers, and spinach.

Cabbage, broccoli, brussels sprouts, kale, and collard greens are also rich in phytochemicals (healing chemicals naturally found in plants) that may inhibit estrogen synthesis and guard you against estrogen overload. In one study, women who ate the most fruits and vegetables were least likely to get breast cancer.

Reach for olive oil. Because it is made up mostly of monounsaturated fat, olive oil doesn't affect your body the way saturated fat (found in animal fats and some plant-based fats such as palm and coconut oil) does. A study of more than 2,000 women in Greece suggests that those who used olive oil more than once a day had a 25 percent lower risk of breast cancer.

Savor soy foods. Soybeans, soy nuts, soy milk, and other soy foods are rich in phytoestrogens, plant chemicals that seem to protect against breast cancer. As these compounds latch on to your body's estrogen receptor cells, they crowd out your body's own estrogen, a suspected "fuel" for breast cancer. Women who live in countries where people eat lots of soy have lower rates of breast cancer.

Eat fatty fish. Substances known as omega-3 fatty acids are found in fish like tuna and salmon. In the laboratory, mice injected with human breast cancer cells developed smaller, less invasive tumors when fed these fatty acids.

Toss in flaxseeds. These tiny edible seeds contain substances called lignans that seem to help fight off breast cancer. Studies at the University of Toronto suggest that flaxseed both inhibits and slows the progression of breast cancer. Grind the seeds in a coffee grinder or food processor for a few seconds so that they're easier to digest. Then sprinkle the seed on your cereal or salad. Flaxseed oil won't do, though; it doesn't contain enough lignan.

Cut out the fat. Population studies show that every country where the diet is low in fat has a low risk of breast cancer, and every country where the diet is high in fat has a high risk. Unfortunately, moderate reductions in fat intake don't seem to help much. Think major cuts.

Fill up with fiber. A high-fiber diet may help the body cleanse itself of excess estrogen. It'll also help you control your weight, because bulky high-fiber food fills you up before you can pack in lots of calories. Weight control is key since body fat actually manufactures a type of estrogen.

Flavor with garlic. This aromatic herb seems to stimulate the immune system. Garlic appears to protect against a wide variety of cancers, including breast cancer.

Make green tea. Asian societies in which women consume a lot of green tea tend to have less breast cancer and less cancer in general. Plant chemicals called polyphenols seem to be responsible. You can also get polyphenols (although in small amounts) in black tea. Look for green tea in your supermarket.

Get out and exercise. When researchers at Arizona State University in Tempe analyzed numerous studies, they found that women who pursued very active jobs, such as teaching physical education, could have up to 50 percent less chance of getting breast cancer than those with sedentary jobs, such as doing office work.

Researchers suggest that moderate physical activity is a deterrent to breast cancer because exercise helps lower weight and body fat, which means that the body is exposed to lower levels of estrogen.

Fibrocystic Changes

Few things in life are as unnerving as feeling a lump or pain in your breast. The good news is most lumps aren't cancerous, and pain is rarely a sign of breast cancer. Normal breast tissue feels lumpy and may feel painful at various points during your menstrual cycle.

Two conditions, fibrocystic breast changes and what doctors call fibroadenoma, are associated with changes in the breast. If you have a fibrocystic condition, your breasts will feel both lumpy and painful before your period. The milk glands in your breasts may enlarge and feel like hard lumps, your breasts' connective tissue may thicken and feel ropy, or the glands may get blocked and filled with fluid, forming cysts.

With a fibroadenoma, your milk glands enlarge, forming a nodule that feels like a solid, rubbery lump. If you have a fibroadenoma, you won't have pain, and the lumpiness won't change over the course of your cycle.

Alternative remedies can help shrink noncancerous lumps and prevent new ones. And various alternatives to prescription and over-the-counter painkillers can help relieve breast tenderness and pain and keep lumps at bay. If your breasts become more tender and swollen after a day or two or they still hurt after 3 months, see your doctor.

Reduce lumps with evening primrose. An effective anti-inflammatory, evening primrose oil can soothe pain and help shrink lumps. Look for evening primrose oil in health food stores, and add a tablespoon of it to your morning oatmeal or sprinkle it over your salad. Or take one or two capsules two or three times a day.

Caution: Don't use evening primrose oil during pregnancy; it may cause miscarriage or premature labor.

Can cola, chocolate, tea, and coffee. Cola, chocolate, tea, and coffee all contain methylxanthines, naturally occurring substances that may contribute to lumpiness and pain.

Brew a cup of herbal tea. Corn silk and buchu, herbal teas found at health food stores, act as mild diuretics that can flush out some of the fluid that contributes to breast discomfort.

Up your fiber. Consume at least 30 grams of fiber a day. Both kinds of fiber, soluble and insoluble, help escort excess estrogen from your body.

Add vitamin E. Some studies have shown that vitamin E—when taken in quantities slightly larger than the recommended daily value—is very effective in relieving breast tenderness and discomfort from fibrocystic breasts. You can start by taking 30 international units (IU) of E a day (that's the recommended daily value) and increasing the amount when you experience breast problems. Or you could simply take 200 to 400 IU of vitamin E every day. But don't take more. Vitamin E is stored in your body fat, so too much could be toxic.

Soothe with vitamin C. When pain and lumpiness are at their worst, try 500 milligrams of vitamin C every couple of hours, for a total daily intake of 3,000 to 5,000 milligrams. Doses this high ease and prevent inflammation. (Excess vitamin C may cause diarrhea in some people.)

Sagging Breasts

Tissues called ligaments hold up the breasts. Unfortunately, they aren't very strong and can lose elasticity with pregnancy, nursing, and age. Although some of these changes are unavoidable, there are steps you can take to keep your breasts on the up-and-up.

Get the right support. A good support bra allows for minimal bounce and puts less stress on your ligaments. The more you wear one during the day, the more it helps. A sports bra, which adds the strongest support, is espe-

The Right Way to Examine Your Breasts

To detect breast cancer in its early, most treatable stages, your doctor should examine your breasts once a year during your routine checkup. But your breasts can change in between yearly visits. So it's important to examine your breasts yourself once a month. Also, if you're over 40, you should talk with your doctor about regular mammograms.

A breast self-exam takes only a few minutes. Here's how to do one.

Start by choosing a date for your monthly self-exam. If you're still menstruating, it's best to perform your self-exam after your monthly period, when your breasts are less likely to be tender or swollen, says Margaret Polaneczky, M.D., assistant professor of obstetrics and gynecology at New York Hospital–Cornell Medical Center in New York City. If you no longer menstruate, choose a date that's easy to remember, like the first of each month. Then follow these steps. If you find a lump, discharge, or any other changes in your breast, see your doctor right away.

1. Stand in front of a mirror with your arms at your sides. Visually check both breasts and nipples for anything unusual, such as puckering, dimpling, or scaliness.
2. Place your hands behind your head and press your hands forward. Look for any change in the shape of your breasts.

cially important if you jog, play tennis, do aerobics, or participate in other forms of exercise.

Push them up. Not with a bra but with a pushup exercise. Exercise won't build up breasts that are already sag-

3. Place your hands on your hips. Push your shoulders and elbows forward and bend toward the mirror. Again, look for any change in the shape of your breasts.
4. Gently squeeze each nipple to check for discharge. Discharge from the bumps around the nipple, known as Montgomery's glands, is totally normal. A little milk or greenish discharge from the nipple itself is not uncommon in women who have had children or who are taking birth control pills. A bloody or clear discharge from the nipple, however, is cause for concern.
5. Raising one arm, use the fingers of your other hand to feel for any fixed, hard, unusual lumps in your breast and the surrounding area, including the armpit area and the region below your collarbone. Be sure to cover the entire surface of your breast, using a specific pattern: lines, circles, or wedges. (Some women find it easier to perform this step in the shower when their skin is soapy.) Repeat on your other breast.
6. Repeat step 5 while lying on your back, with one arm over your head and a pillow under your shoulder. This is a position that flattens out the breast, making it easier to feel for lumps.

ging, because breast tissue is mostly fat. But this pushup will build up the pectoral muscle underneath, which will make your breasts look perkier.

Lie on your stomach with your hands next to your chest. Straighten your arms and push up your torso, keeping your head aligned with your torso, your back straight, and your knees on the floor. Slowly return to your starting position. Aim for three sets of 12 repetitions each. Rest for 1½ minutes between sets.

Start to fly. To build more muscle, try what's called the dumbbell fly, using a pair of 1- to 3-pound weights.

To start, pick up one weight in each hand, then lie on your back on a carpeted floor or an exercise mat. Extend your arms out on the floor at shoulder level, with your palms up, clutching your weights. The weights should be parallel to your body. Draw both arms straight up together above your body, keeping your elbows slightly bent, so that the weights meet over your chest. Then return the weights to your sides at shoulder height, as if you were drawing a semicircle or half-moon over your body. Repeat the exercise 12 to 15 times, then rest for 1½ minutes. Do three sets, resting between sets.

The stronger you become, the more weight you'll be able to handle. This means you should be able to gradually increase the weights you use by 1 or 2 pounds. As you use heavier weights, decrease the number of repetitions you do, aiming for 8 to 10 repetitions per set. Continue to do three sets.

Rub on sun protection. Sun exposure can speed up the aging of elastin fibers that keep your skin from sagging. So make sure that you apply sunscreen to your chest area whenever you wear a sundress, tank top, or bathing suit with a low neckline. Many dermatologists recommend a sun protection factor (SPF) of 15. Whatever you use, don't forget to reapply it regularly.

Bra Problems

Bras can chafe, irritate the skin, or let you down when you need support the most—especially if you're large-breasted. But your bra doesn't have to sentence you to a lifetime of discomfort. By taking a few commonsense steps, you can find comfort and support in this vital undergarment.

Test-drive your bra. To make sure that a bra fits, always try it on before you buy it. The cups should completely contain your breasts, with no bulges at the tops or sides of the cups. The bra should be loose enough for you to slip a finger under the band at the base of the cups. If there are wrinkles in the cups, it means the bra is too large. Also, make sure that the bra doesn't ride up in the back. If it does, the bra may be too large or hooked too loosely, or the straps may be too tight.

Check inside the cups for seams that may chafe. If there is an underwire, make sure that it is very well padded so that it doesn't add to the friction.

Search for thickness. Large-breasted women should buy bras with thick straps, which support the breasts better and do not cut into the shoulders. For the same effect, you can also buy strap pads and attach them yourself.

Sport the right bra. If you're a C cup or larger and in the market for a sports bra, look for one with good support that controls your breast movement. Some women find that nonelastic shoulder straps are best for minimizing movement. Sports bras are available in the lingerie departments of some department stores and in sporting goods stores.

Rise a size. Wear a larger-size bra when your breasts hurt. Select one that keeps your breasts secure without being uncomfortably constricting. A sports bra with a wide elastic band may be your best bet.

Take it off. If your bra has chafed your skin, ease the irritation by going braless at home. Pull on a caftan or loose shirt that allows air to circulate freely around your breasts.

Soothe them with calendula cream. If your breasts are chafed and irritated, smooth on a healing cream made with the herb calendula. Researchers have found that calendula extracts can decrease swelling and increase skin-healing activity. They're antiseptic too. Look for calendula cream in health food stores.

Try aloe vera. Snip a leaf from the easy-to-grow aloe vera plant on your windowsill, slit it open, and scoop out the cool, clear gel that's inside. Smooth it on chafed skin for cooling relief.

No-Pause Menopause

For a woman, menopause is aging's main event.

Physically, her body undergoes significant changes—her periods come to an end and hormone levels decline, often causing a range of discomforts such as hot flashes and vaginal dryness.

Mentally, she experiences emotional ups and downs that come with surging hormones and the knowledge that the body that she has been familiar with for some 40 years is forever changing.

Spiritually, she faces new possibilities and challenges as she exits her childbearing years for things unknown.

All told, many women say that these multiple changes are a good thing.

"Menopause is positive if you make it positive," says Helen Healy, N.D., a naturopathic physician and owner and director of the Wellspring Naturopathic Clinic in St. Paul, Minnesota. "Many women feel free and glad that they don't have to be concerned with monthly periods anymore."

Officially, you haven't "arrived" at menopause until

you've gone 1 full year without a period. While it's different for every woman, this usually happens sometime after age 50. But you may begin noticing signs of this approaching transition in your early forties—or even in your mid-thirties.

During this period of very gradual change, called perimenopause, a woman's supply of the female hormone estrogen starts to waver, which can create some of the same problems women get in the throes of menopause—hot flashes, vaginal dryness, mood swings, and sleeping problems. Of course, not everyone has such discomfort: One in three women sails through menopause symptom-free.

The biggest negative of menopause is that it leaves you open to some serious health problems. That's because estrogen is a natural fortress against heart disease, bone loss, and breast cancer. To compensate for the loss of estrogen, many doctors today recommend hormone replacement therapy (HRT).

Easing into Menopause

Whether to take HRT is a decision you should make in consultation with your doctor. Sometimes, natural treatments such as herbs, exercise, healing foods, and vitamins can be just as effective as HRT for relieving symptoms of menopause, says Dr. Healy. "If you can do what women did in the past—which was exercise a lot, eat well, and use herbs—you may not even need to take hormones at all," she says. Here are some natural healing ideas for the menopause years.

Combine some herbs. An herbal product specifically formulated for menopause may help lessen hormone-related discomforts such as hot flashes and mood swings. Such a product usually contains some combination of the following herbs: chasteberry (sometimes called vitex), black cohosh, dong quai, panax ginseng (sometimes called Asian ginseng), and licorice root.

You will find these herbal blends in health food stores. Look for a product that contains standardized extracts. A

The Natural Route to Hormone Replacement

When the time comes to consider hormone replacement therapy, consider "going natural," says Connie Catellani, M.D., medical director at the Miro Center for Integrative Medicine in Evanston, Illinois.

Choose one of the plant-based progesterone creams available in health food stores. The progesterone in natural progesterone creams (sold under brand names including NatraGest and Pro-Gest) has a molecular structure identical to that of the body's own "homemade" progesterone. The result is fewer side effects.

In contrast, synthetic hormone supplements—sold under brand names including Premarin and Provera—have a molecular "shape" slightly different from that produced by the body. These forms are more potent and last longer and can cause more side effects, Dr. Catellani says.

It's important to note that both natural and synthetic hormone supplements are made in pharmaceutical laboratories from sources including wild yams and soybeans (and, in the case of Premarin, from the urine of pregnant horses). "The natural products are natural because of their structure, not because of their origins," Dr. Catellani notes.

standardized extract is guaranteed to contain a specific amount of an herb's active ingredient.

Note: Dong quai causes some people to become more sensitive to the sun. If you choose a product containing this herb, be especially cautious when you head outdoors. Also, if you choose a product containing licorice root, do not use it for more than 6 weeks, and avoid its use if you have diabetes, high blood pressure, or a liver or kidney disorder.

Eat grazefully. Eating small meals 2 to 3 hours apart may help you avoid menopausal weight gain.

Watch your cholesterol. Estrogen seems to protect a woman's heart by keeping cholesterol levels in line. After menopause, women have higher levels of artery-clogging low-density lipoprotein (LDL) cholesterol and lower levels of artery-cleaning high-density lipoprotein (HDL) cholesterol.

Studies show that limiting fat to 25 to 30 percent of your daily calories will help keep the bad guys under control.

Stay active. Research has proven that regular exercise helps combat weight gain, heart disease, and osteoporosis—problems that a woman is more likely to experience following menopause.

So start walking, swimming, biking, rowing, or jogging. Take an aerobics class (or pop an aerobics video into your home VCR). Any activity that elevates your heart rate will help.

Chat with your partner. Open communication with your significant other is especially important now. Share your menopausal experiences and thoughts, and the two of you will grow closer. It's especially important to address physical changes that can impact shared activities, such as vaginal dryness that can make sex uncomfortable or hot flashes that might leave you a little distracted.

Keep your B and C up. Take 1,000 milligrams of vitamin C and 50 milligrams of B-complex vitamins twice each day. (Make sure your B-complex supplement contains pantothenic acid.) These vitamins support your adrenal glands, tiny powerhouses on top of your kidneys that continue to produce small amounts of estrogen.

Note: Some people experience diarrhea when they take more than 1,000 milligrams of vitamin C a day. If this happens to you, simply reduce your intake of the vitamin until the diarrhea subsides.

Fill up on fennel. Eat at least one serving (about ½ cup) of Umbelliferae each day. This group of plants—which includes fennel, parsley, and celery—contains phytoestrogens, compounds with estrogen-like activity.

Bone Protection

Getting enough calcium—from food and supplements—is especially important for women approaching menopause. Without enough calcium, your skeleton can grow weak when estrogen levels fall because this hormone helps bones absorb and retain calcium, the main component of bone. In fact, the highest rate of bone loss occurs in the first 5 to 7 years after menopause.

The good news is that osteoporosis is often preventable. In one study, researchers in the Netherlands found that women who consumed at least 1,000 milligrams of calcium a day—the amount found in about three 8-ounce glasses of milk—were able to reduce bone loss by 43 percent.

Before menopause, aim for 1,000 milligrams of calcium a day. During and after menopause, you need 1,200 to 1,500 milligrams of this important bone-maintaining mineral daily. Try these easy and flavorful ways to get more calcium into your diet.

Sip low-fat and fat-free milk. Don't overlook milk, even if you're trying to cut calories by consuming less fat. Low-fat and fat-free versions have significantly less fat and calories than whole milk and, glass for glass, provide more calcium because manufacturers replace some of the fat with extra calcium.

Sprinkle on the cheese. Just like milk, many cheeses now come in low-fat and fat-free versions. One-half cup of ricotta has 337 milligrams of calcium. One tablespoon of low-fat Parmesan provides almost 70 milligrams of calcium.

Powder your baked goods. Add nonfat dry milk to baked goods like muffins and cakes. One-half cup of fat-free milk powder contains almost 420 milligrams of calcium.

Power up your breakfast. When making hot cereal such as oatmeal, substitute 1 cup of low-fat milk for the cooking water, then add ½ cup of milk powder to the finished cereal. This one-two punch delivers 720 milligrams of calcium.

Pour a glass of OJ. Dairy isn't the only source of calcium anymore. Many brands of orange juice and other juices have been fortified and have as much calcium as a glass of milk.

Get a surprise calcium boost—from greens. Help yourself to kale, broccoli, collards, and turnip greens. These greens contain 36 to 94 milligrams of calcium per cup—enough to help you meet your daily needs.

Serve up salmon. Try canned pink salmon *with* the bones. Thanks to the tiny bones, 3 ounces of the fish contains about 180 milligrams of calcium.

Take the right supplement. While food can supply ample amounts of calcium, it's difficult to consume 1,000 to 1,500 milligrams of calcium each and every day from edibles alone. And it's impossible to cram that much calcium into a multivitamin and mineral tablet. So doctors recommend that women take a separate calcium supplement.

Which one? Read the labels. The best (and least expensive) contain calcium carbonate. These provide the highest percentage of calcium and are well-absorbed when taken with food.

For enhanced absorption, add vitamin D. Choose a daily multivitamin or calcium supplement that contains 400 international units of vitamin D, the vitamin that supports bone maintenance by helping your body absorb calcium.

Maximize magnesium. This vital mineral helps your bones absorb calcium and converts vitamin D into its active form in your body. Excellent food sources of magnesium include almonds, toasted wheat germ, seafood, low-fat cheeses, broccoli, baked potatoes, and bananas. Aim for 400 milligrams a day, from food plus a magnesium-containing supplement if necessary.

Exercise against gravity. Weight-bearing exercises—which include cardiovascular activities such as walking, running, aerobics, and racquet sports as well as weight lifting—can also help build bone mass. Aim for three or four 30-minute sessions a week.

Hot Flashes

Of all the changes heralding menopause, most women agree that the hot flash is the most notorious. Happily, most research into natural remedies for menopause has focused on this symptom.

Starting as a sudden warmth in your face, head, or chest, a hot flash can spread like wildfire in just seconds. Then, as your body tries to cool itself off, you sweat. The kicker to a reddening, drenching hot flash can be a bout of shivering chills as your body reacts to your wide-open pores and dampened skin.

If you're among the estimated 75 to 85 percent of women who experience hot flashes, try these time-tested natural strategies for relief, offered by alternative practitioners.

Take a deep breath. In one study, women who had experienced 20 or more hot flashes a day reduced that number by half with the help of deep breathing.

When you feel a hot flash creeping up on you, prepare for deep breathing by sitting up straight and loosening your belt or waistband if it feels tight. Begin by exhaling through your nose longer than you normally would. Then inhale through your nose slowly and deeply, filling your lungs from the bottom up while keeping your belly relaxed. When your chest is fully expanded, exhale slowly and deeply, as if sighing. Continue until the hot flash subsides.

Cool with black cohosh. Black cohosh has been shown to be as effective as estrogen for the relief of hot flashes. You may need to use it for up to 4 weeks before you feel better, however.

To find the best dosage, start by taking 10 drops of black cohosh tincture (also known as an extract) in a small amount of water or juice twice a day. Then increase the dose by 5 drops every other day until you are satisfied with the results.

Some women take black cohosh daily. Others take it simply when needed. Some women find relief by taking it for 2 consecutive weeks each month. Experiment to see what works best for you, but don't take it for more than 6 months, for it could have some side effects such as diarrhea, abdominal pain, and headache.

Start a bath. Before going to bed, draw a comfortably warm—not hot—bath. Then soak in it long enough for the water to cool, which should take about 20 minutes. This bedtime ritual may interrupt a pattern of night sweats (nocturnal hot flashes) so that they occur less frequently and are less severe.

To enhance the therapeutic effects of your bath, add the following essential oils: 4 drops of chamomile, 6 drops of lemon, and 10 drops of evening primrose. Chamomile is said to relax the body, while lemon cools and evening primrose aids hormonal balance. You can buy essential oils in health food stores.

Adjust your thermostat. If you can, adjust the temperature of the room you are in to 60°F. Simplistic as it may seem, turning down the heat or cranking up the air-conditioning is solid advice. Anything that raises body temperature even a tiny bit can aggravate a hot flash.

Skip hot spices. Hot tamales or curried chicken may taste great, but such foods tend to trigger hot flashes.

Cut back on caffeine. Caffeine is a stimulant and can trigger hot flashes by raising your blood pressure and heart rate.

Sip some ice water. Minimize the inconvenience of nighttime hot flashes by keeping a carafe of ice water on your night table.

Dress in layers. Stay comfortable by slipping off clothes as your body temperature rises.

Mood Swings

It's not clear whether menopause *causes* mood disorders, but it may make existing moodiness more apparent. Some women's emotions seem to be particularly sensitive to hormonal changes at midlife. For them, menopause may unmask mild depression, irritability, memory problems, and even sleep disturbances. Here are some options to control your swinging moods.

Relax. In the midst of a bad mood, try a relaxation technique that appeals to you. Some doctors recommend relaxing exercises such as yoga and meditation. Other tactics that may be helpful include deep breathing, visualization, and exercise.

Soothe with skullcap. Skullcap herbal tincture (available in health food stores) strengthens the nerves, eases

Why Women Grow Shorter

As we age, the density of our bones begins breaking down faster than new bone can be formed. It's common for some women to lose ½ to 1 inch in height because of normal degenerative changes in the spine. Anything more than that should be cause for concern.

Loss of height is often the first sign of osteoporosis, a condition in which bones get thinner and brittle, says Kendra Zuckerman, M.D., assistant professor of medicine and associate director of clinical programs at the Osteoporosis and Bone Metabolism Center at Allegheny University Hospital in Philadelphia. While osteoporosis strikes both men and women, it develops a lot faster and at a younger age in women, in large part because of the sudden drop in estrogen—a hormone that has protected women's bones all their lives—following menopause.

In its early stages, osteoporosis is painless and, outside of a little shrinking, offers no visible signs. In fact, it's usually a broken bone that sends up the red flag. In late stages of the disease, a woman can lose up to 4 to 8 inches of height and develop the classic dowager's hump. By this time, she'll frequently have pain.

Once lost, bone density is difficult to replace—and so osteoporosis is difficult to treat. That's why it's important to prevent it through weight-bearing exercise and a diet that includes plenty of calcium.

oversensitivity, and helps promote deep, sound sleep. Take four to eight drops of the tincture mornings and evenings in a small glass of water or juice if you're feeling stressed-out or just wound up. (Do not confuse it with Chinese skullcap, which has entirely different properties.)

Take a quick walk. When bad moods occur during low-energy periods, moderate exercise can help. Don't walk so fast that you become exhausted—just fast enough to become energized.

Eat. Don't skip meals. As with PMS-related mood swings, missed meals and dieting can affect your moods.

Vaginal Dryness

As estrogen levels dwindle, the lining of your vagina may become drier, thinner, and less flexible. You may notice such changes most during sex—you're aroused, but you're not as lushly lubricated as you used to be. As a result, sexual intercourse can be painful or even impossible.

While vaginal dryness poses no serious threat to your health, it can be a barrier to intimacy. Here are some self-care solutions.

Bring out the sesame oil. Some women report having great success using sesame oil to relieve vaginal dryness. Soak a Coets (quilted cotton cosmetic square) in sesame oil, squeeze out the excess oil, insert it into the vagina, and leave it in overnight. Remove the Coets the next morning, and that night, replace it with a new one also dipped in sesame oil. Repeat every day for a week, then once a week for as long as necessary. The sesame oil may induce an estrogen-like effect.

Try a homeopathic lubricant. For relief from menopause-related vaginal dryness, try a vaginal suppository containing vitamin E and a beeswax base. Begin by using one suppository every night for 6 weeks, then cut back to one suppository one night a week for as long as needed. You can buy vitamin E suppositories in health food stores.

Chew on licorice root. Chew two tablets (a total of 380 milligrams) of deglycyrrhizinated licorice root about 30 minutes before each meal. Licorice root targets vaginal dryness in two ways. For starters, the herb stimulates mucus production in your body, even increasing the number of goblet cells (cells that manufacture mucus). Plus, licorice root contains compounds that act as weak forms of estrogen. You can buy chewable tablets of deglycyrrhizinated licorice root in health food stores. ("Deglycyrrhizinated—DGL" means that the compounds in licorice that elevate blood pressure have been removed.)

Return to the essentials. If your vagina is parched, you may be deficient in essential fatty acids, oils found in plants and fish that are essential to the health of, among other things, vaginal tissues. Help lubricate your vagina by ingesting a tablespoon of fatty acid–rich flaxseed oil daily.

Use vitamin E every day. Take 400 international units of vitamin E each day. Traditionally, research has paid little attention to the effects of this vitamin on vaginal dryness though evidence of its power has been around for some time. Two studies done in the 1940s indicate that vitamin E supplements can improve symptoms of vaginal atrophy. If you decide to try it, give yourself at least 4 weeks to see results.

Carry a water bottle. Drink at least eight 8-ounce glasses of water or fresh juice each day. Even mild dehydration—the kind that is barely noticeable to most people—can dry out mucous membranes in the vagina.

Part Four

Your Mind

Master Your Moods

Blue Mondays. In a funk. Down in the dumps. Bored to tears.

"Moods are our bodies' barometers as we react to different situations going on around us or within us," says Leah Dickstein, M.D., professor and director of the division of attitudinal and behavioral medicine in the department of psychiatry at the University of Louisville School of Medicine in Kentucky.

Managing your moods can help you get on with your life with your customary energy, determination, and enthusiasm, says Dr. Dickstein.

To achieve your best, here's how you can learn to control your moods—even learn from them.

Anger

Everyone gets angry. Not everyone goes ballistic, however. And how you react when you are angry determines whether your response is either toxic or constructive to your health and to others.

Think of anger as hot sauce bubbling in a pot on the stove. If you put a lid on it, it will boil over. Similarly, seething until you boil over can raise your blood pressure or contribute to heart disease. If you throw a tantrum or say things that you will regret, you can alienate others, like your husband, your friends, or your boss.

"Anger is healthy as long as you're not physical and hurt others or yourself," says Dr. Dickstein. The key is learning to express your anger. Here's how.

Freeze. The instant you feel your pulse quicken with anger, don't speak or move for a moment. This silent pause gives you time to think about the situation and handle it constructively.

Inhale the scent of roses. Take a whiff of rose oil, considered by aromatherapists to be the classic remedy for anger. Place a couple drops of essential oil of rose on a handkerchief and inhale the scent for 1 to 3 minutes. Look for essential oils in health food stores.

Deal with issues, not personalities. Don't focus on blaming whoever made you angry. The other person will stop listening and get defensive, blocking a solution. Instead, frame your response with solution-seeking phrases such as "Let's look at the situation a different way" or "This doesn't seem fair. What can we do to improve the situation?"

Bad Moods

A scowl is chiseled into your face. Your spouse and kids stay out of your way. The cat dives for cover. Diagnosis: You are in a bad mood.

Bad moods are more than one emotion rolled into one—usually anger, anxiety, and depression. The following remedies work on more than one emotional layer at a time.

Who's Moodier—Men or Women?

Females take the rap for being the moodier of the sexes, and it's fueled by the belief that the ups and downs of their hormone levels are linked to the ups and downs of their moods.

While it's true that some women tend to get crankier at a certain time of the month, females by no means take the gold when it comes to the moody blues.

Moodiness actually strikes both genders about equally and has a lot to do with how a person looks at life, says Susan Olson, Ph.D., a clinical psychologist in Seattle.

People who are moody often feel a lack of control over their lives, says Dr. Olson. They may assume they are somehow at fault when things don't go well, or they may have the underlying expectation that the world owes them something.

"Moody people can get stuck on a negative thought and generalize it to other things," Dr. Olson adds. "For example, they could say to themselves, 'I didn't do this well. I never do anything right.'"

Gender, however, does seem to have some bearing on how people behave during a mood swing. "In my observation, men are less likely to handle their moods as openly and emotionally as women. Men may appear more angry or withdrawn, whereas many women openly express their feelings of sadness with tears," explains Dr. Olson.

Walk it off. A 20-to-30-minute brisk walk, jog, or bike ride—anything that gets your heart pumping and works up a sweat—triggers the release of endorphins, mood-enhancing chemicals produced by the brain.

Breathe and jot. Find a quiet spot, and take deep, meditative breaths until you feel your heart rate and pulse slow down. Write down what has you in a bad mood. Then take action to undo whatever brought on the bad mood.

"If you're mad at yourself, tell yourself, 'I'm learning something about what I did wrong, and I will try not to let it happen again. It's the best I can do,'" says Dr. Dickstein.

Grin and share it. Sometimes, simply smiling at yourself or others can lift you out of a bad mood. So if you are feeling cranky, head for the nearest mirror and give yourself a big smile.

Sidestep touchy topics or touchy people. Bad moods can be contagious and spread their irritability and anger quickly. When you are in a bad mood, avoid topics, activities, or people that you know spark discord.

Turn off the TV. Vegging in front of the television is the worst way to fend off a bad mood. Staring at the screen prolongs grouchiness and does nothing to improve matters.

The Blues

A case of the blues is the common cold of emotional health. Instead of sniffling, you weep. Instead of running a fever, you mope. Instead of coughing, you sit in silence. As with a cold, you could wait out the blues. Or you could try to conquer them on your own with these remedies.

Take some B_6. If the blues seem to stem from premenstrual syndrome (PMS), take 25 to 50 milligrams of vitamin B_6 daily. Two out of three women who try this find that it improves their moods by their next menstrual cycle.

Strike up the band. Music lifts your spirits by altering levels of stress hormones in your blood, which in turn slows down your breathing and heart rate. Keep a special stash of mood-elevating CDs on hand to conquer your next blue mood.

Draw, color, or paint. If you are upset, creating anything artistic can lift you out of a bad mood. Keep a stash of crayons and drawing paper handy. Or make a collage out of magazine photos and glue.

Boredom

Variety keeps your brain stimulated and your body refreshed and energized. Sameness, on the other hand, is like "mental fat"—mental and physical sluggishness that can leave you dissatisfied with yourself or others, unproductive, even angry. Worse, boredom can lead to overeating or bad habits like smoking and drinking. Here are healthier ways to punch up your life.

Give yourself a new job. Whenever that "same-old, same-old" feeling creeps into your work, it's likely you're ready for more challenges. Volunteer for a special assignment or ask your boss for new and different responsibilities. Apply for a new job within your company. Or polish your résumé and look for a job elsewhere.

Tackle a dream. Nothing stimulates your brain like learning. Make a list of things you always wished you could do—fix a leaky faucet, speak a foreign language, or do photography. Then call the local community college and enroll in a noncredit class in whatever subject interests you.

Go from passive to passionate. Maybe you already have plenty of hobbies, but they are getting a little routine. Ratchet up to the next level. Love to read murder mysteries? Don't just read books. Attend a murder mystery dinner-theater performance, where the audience sorts through clues to find out "whodunit" and why.

Recruit an adventure buddy. If your spouse or best friend is equally bored, tackle adventure together. Put together a 3-D puzzle. Complete a 50-mile bike ride for charity. Join a crew building a house for Habitat for Humanity. No takers? Plunge ahead on your own.

Depression

You can't get out of bed. Or you can't sleep. You can't eat. Or you overeat. Or you are sad, empty, or anxious, and it just won't let up.

Mild depression often manifests itself as deeply negative feelings of sorrow, guilt, discouragement, and powerlessness. If you have mild depression, the following home remedies may help. If, however, depression is interfering with your life—if you have trouble concentrating or lose interest in your normal activities—or your depression interferes with your job, see a doctor.

Pick up some St. John's wort. Fast becoming the herb of choice of Americans with bouts of mild depression, St. John's wort supplements work with your body's brain chemistry to elevate mood and ease fatigue without the side effects of prescription medications such as fluoxetine (Prozac).

Note: If you are already on antidepressant medication, take this herb only with your doctor's supervision.

Turn in your M&Ms. People who are mildly depressed seem to crave sweets constantly. The refined sugar found in candies and cakes offers a fast mood fix, but the effect is short-lived. Your blood sugar level quickly dives, leaving you feeling down or, in some cases, even more miserable and tired.

Try fighting the sugar blues by eating more foods with complex carbohydrates. Foods like rice cakes, corn on the cob, oatmeal, and English muffins boost your levels of the natural feel-good chemical serotonin and help you relax.

Seek the sun. If you get depressed and listless during the dark winter months, take a 30-minute walk at daybreak every day, even if it is cold. Increasing your exposure to daylight during the winter months helps you avoid seasonal affective disorder (SAD), a condition that is common in the winter and causes depression, mood and appetite changes, and a tendency to withdraw and to sleep a lot.

Best Stress Defense

On any given day, the average person plays any one of dozens of possible roles: Parent. Child. Spouse. Employee. Employer. Committee chair. Good neighbor. Volunteer. Cook. Housekeeper. Dog walker. The list goes on.

It all adds up to too much responsibility, too little control, and too little time—the perfect formula for stress overload.

In the world of emotions, stress is the big mama to anxiety, burnout, nervous tension, and worry. Collectively or separately, these emotions can be powerful enemies to the joys we seek in life.

A little stress, of course, is healthy. It can challenge and energize. But too much for too long can pummel your immune system and cause physical symptoms, such as muscle aches, headaches, rapid heartbeat, elevated blood pressure, and irritability.

"Stress is a fact of life. There's no such thing as a life without stress," says psychologist Susan Jeffers, Ph.D., author of *End the Struggle and Dance with Life*. It only becomes a problem when we can't cope with it.

"The best way to cope with stress is to learn how to let go and trust you will handle whatever happens in your life," says Dr. Jeffers. "And stop trying to be perfect. Even the Buddha had bad days."

10 Natural Stress Busters

Experts like Dr. Jeffers say that it's best to relax *before* you implode. If you're stressed day in and day out, your body actually forgets what it's like to feel calm. To build resiliency, try the following.

Take a breather. Make time for regular relaxation breaks in the day—once or twice a day for 10 minutes.

Inhale and exhale slowly. While watching a scary scene in a movie, you naturally hold your breath or breathe too shallowly. It's an automatic fright reaction by your body's defense system. The same thing happens when you feel anxious.

Keeping this in mind, try to focus first on your breathing the next time you feel tense for any reason. Take slow, deep breaths that come from deep inside your diaphragm, located just below your rib cage. To make sure that you're breathing correctly, place your open palm on your diaphragm. Your hand should rise every time you inhale and drop every time you exhale.

As you become accustomed to this breathing pattern, you may want to whisper a word such as *relax* or *calm* as you exhale.

Conjure up a soothing image. Picture yourself lounging on a tropical beach or in a hammock under your favorite tree—anything that makes you feel calm and peaceful. Be sure to include all your senses—the smells of the ocean or leaves, heat of the sun, coolness of a breeze, taste of a pineapple or lemonade.

Sweat stress away. Any activity that gets you moving—such as walking, swimming, tennis, and jogging—generates feel-good brain chemicals known as endorphins while helping to burn off stress-related chemicals like adrenaline, especially if you do the activity for at least 30 minutes four or five times a week.

Prioritize your time. When you find yourself faced with a plateful of tasks, ask yourself, "What's necessary and what's not?" Then do what you must, and let the rest go.

Cluster tasks. You may be wasting precious time and not even realize it. For 7 days, write down every 15 minutes what you are doing. Review the log at the end of the week. Then try to group errands or delete unnecessary activities.

Know when to say, "Good enough." Trying to do an A-plus job at every task, no matter how big or how small, creates a second helping of stress. If you tend to strive for perfection, try lowering your expectations a bit. Know when B work is acceptable, and give yourself permission to adjust accordingly. Your nerves will thank you.

Speak up. When you are stressed because you feel powerless over your obligations and responsibilities, speak up. Faced with too many assignments at work—or too many household chores—you feel overloaded and taxed to the max. So say something. Review your workload with your boss. Let your family know that they're not doing their share. Then divide the work equitably. Others may not realize that you're overloaded.

Take an aromatherapy bath. To defuse a pressure-filled day, soak in a hot bath sprinkled with essential oils, scents favored by aromatherapists for their stress-busting potential. For stress-induced moodiness or depression, add one to five drops of geranium oil to your bathwater. For an emotional lift, try a few drops of essential oil of sweet orange in your bath.

Get off the more-better-best treadmill. All the tension-taming tricks in the world are powerless against stress unless you develop a stress-resilient philosophy. Constant striving for more of anything—money, position, status, possessions, awards, accomplishments—can become addictive and leave you physically and mentally stressed.

To step off this escalator, redefine success. Concentrate on process, not results: tending a small garden instead of maintaining a big house, reading to your children instead of competing for yet another promotion.

Anxiety

Anxiety is the emotional phantom of the unknown. It's that vague feeling of dread swirling in the pit of your stomach when you're about to answer the phone in the middle of the night, when your boss says she needs to speak to you, or when your doctor calls you in to follow up on your mammogram. You're not sure what's about to happen, but you don't expect good news.

If not kept in check, anxiety can raise your blood pressure and heart rate and may trigger stomachaches, restlessness, dizziness, and poor concentration. When anxiety is ongoing or so intense that you can't concentrate, sleep, or enjoy yourself, you need relief. If you suffer from these symptoms, see your doctor.

Kick in logic. When anxiety appears, call on logic to come to the rescue. If you catch yourself thinking, "I just don't have the nerve to ask for a raise," stop yourself. Replace that irrational thought with encouraging self-talk such as "I'm a solid worker who has taken extra classes to improve my job skills, and I merit higher pay." Positive self-talk can reduce your anxiety.

Try some kava kava. Experts say that this herb is a safe and natural alternative to sedating, addictive prescription drugs such as alprazolam (Xanax). Available in the form of tablets or liquid extracts, kava kava contains kavalactones and, in low doses, relaxes without the sedating side effects of drugs. In higher doses, kava kava actually acts as a mild sedative to help you sleep. For anxiety relief, experts suggest limiting doses to 70 to 210 milligrams of kavalactones daily.

Take a bath with lavender oil. To calm anxiety and help you get a good night's sleep, aromatherapists suggest that you add a few drops of lavender to your bath.

Apply acupressure. Millions of Chinese rely on acupressure—a variation of acupuncture, without the needles—to relieve stress-related complaints such as anxiety. A quick way to relieve minor anxiety is to apply pressure to the Spirit Gate point, located on the outside of your wrist, below the first crease and in line with your pinkie finger. Press on this spot until you get an aching sensation similar to when you hit your funny bone.

Maintain this pressure for 15 to 30 seconds, then release. For optimum results, do not work the same spot more than two or three times a day.

Burnout

The math never adds up in your favor. It seems that you have too much to do in too little time, with too few resources—a classic case of burnout. Whether it involves your job, your home life, or both, the typical symptoms of burnout are the same: exhaustion, insomnia, hopelessness, and an I-don't-care-anymore attitude.

If you need help, ask for it. You don't have to be all things to everyone 24 hours a day. When tasks start stacking up, speak up. At home, ask for help from family members or friends. If you're juggling a full-time job with caring for teenage children and elderly parents, ask a friend or relative to step in one afternoon or evening to help you out. Do the same at work and enlist help from others on staff.

Set aside 1 hour every day to exercise. When it comes to remedies for stress, you can't get much more natural than exercise. Working out releases endorphins, natural mood-elevating substances in your brain that dissolve tension. Pick a time—either the morning or after work—that suits you best. Don't let family or job responsibilities interrupt this hour. Select a comfortable, convenient place to exercise—whether it's a fitness center, a local park, or even your basement.

Celebrate small victories. Instead of waiting for others to encourage you or give you a pat on the back for accomplishing your goals, rely on yourself for rewards. Treat yourself with a bestseller, a movie, or an iced cappuccino after you meet a deadline.

Turn off technology. Thanks to cellular phones, e-mail, voice mail, and laptop computers, you're never out of reach from your office and your work responsibilities. Resist the temptation to routinely contact the office outside regular business hours. Otherwise, you'll be a perpetual slave to the demands of the job, with no downtime.

Nervous Tension

A nagging, unsettling feeling of unease, nervous tension is first cousin to anxiety. And like anxiety, nervous tension is usually a sign that something you must deal with is bothering you. Outwardly, nervous tension may leave you with a quivering voice, a perspiring face, or shaky hands. Inside your body, this emotion can cause back pain, headaches, stomachaches, and sleepless nights.

Even folks who are normally confident and composed can sometimes get rattled when things go wrong. Here's what to do.

Create an action plan. The first day back at work after a vacation is prime time for nervous tension. Instead of worrying about how you're going to catch up, get out your calendar. Set priorities. Then systematically attack each item, starting with the most urgent or important.

Exercise tension away. This all-purpose tension tamer is made to order for nervous tension. A 30-minute aerobic workout activates endorphins, your brain's feel-good army of chemicals. As the endorphins filter through your body, they provide a sense of well-being and calm. When you feel nervous tension seizing control, counter that by doing an activity you enjoy—perhaps cycling, running, walking, or swimming.

Shun refined sugar. You might be tempted to reach for a cookie or candy bar when nervous tension mounts. Though a sugary treat may appear to be your calming lifeline, its impact is short-lived. Immediately after eating a sugary treat, your blood sugar spikes, making you feel better—temporarily. But within an hour, your blood sugar levels plummet, along with your mood, making you feel even more drained and anxious. Instead, eat whole wheat bread or a slice of turkey breast. Complex carbohydrates and protein provide slow but steady energy that keeps you on an even keel.

Performance Anxiety

You don't have to be an actor to experience performance anxiety. Anyone can experience "stage fright" at home, at work, or at everyday events. You put off calling the new neighbor. You dread being asked to speak at church. You need to make an important business call or have a job interview.

Here's some help for mastering your next presentation or talk.

Prepare—then prepare some more. If you know your material cold, you're less apt to go blank, and you won't have to spend a lot of time or energy trying to remember it under stressful circumstances.

Rehearse, rehearse, rehearse. Keep practicing your role until it feels natural and automatic. That way, when you step up to the podium or walk into the meeting room, you'll feel more confident about being successful in your performance.

Tell yourself it's okay to be nervous. A small case of stage jitters before speaking or making a presentation is normal and healthy. Even some veteran actors admit they're a bit anxious before a performance. So you're in good company!

Visualize a positive outcome. Cognitive therapy is a quick and easy way to prevent nervous tension from making you assume the worst about a situation. Let's say you're a bundle of nerves about facing your first job interview in years. Instead of convincing yourself that you'll mess up during the interview or that people probably won't like you, inject some positive reality into your thoughts.

Walk into the interview with this thought: "Lots of people are nervous during job interviews. It's natural. She interviews hundreds of nervous applicants, so she's used to it and probably won't hold that against me. Besides, they called me right after they got my résumé, so there is something about me that interests them."

Ignore early tremors. If you start out sounding a little nervous, ignore it. Once you get started, performance anxiety usually subsides.

Worry

Face it. Many of us are worriers. We even agonize over circumstances that haven't yet occurred or might never occur.

The symptom is a vocabulary with a long list of what-ifs: What if I miss my deadline? What if I lose my job? What if she misses the plane? What if she can't find her ticket? What if it rains?

We seem to worry most when we're under stress because stress reduces our ability to reason. But experts say that you can reduce the amount of time you spend fretting.

Weed out negative thoughts. When you come right down to it, worry is a bad habit. So replace the bad habit with a good habit. When you catch yourself beginning phrases with "What if" or "I should have," stop and replace them with more positive phrases such as "I can."

Book worry time. Schedule 20 to 30 minutes each day to brood and wonder. This classic antiworry technique gives you time to explore the what-if and if-only thoughts filling your head.

Experts advise that it's best to spend this worrying time in a quiet place where you won't be interrupted. When a worrisome thought pops in your head during the day, jot it down and remind yourself to focus on it during your worry time. Try to avoid booking time right before you go to sleep; otherwise, the worry could intrude on your night's rest.

Consider the worst. To put your worries in perspective, think through each possible scenario and consider what you would do *if* your worries became a reality. Let's say you worry that you'll lose your job. Ask yourself if you would also lose your home. Your family. Never find another job. After listing what might happen, identify ways to deal with each of these specific issues. Then let them go.

Help others. It's a known fact that the more time you devote to helping others, the less time you spend fretting about your own troubles—real or imagined. Consider volunteering as a reading tutor at a local school or as a museum tour guide. Or train to run a 5-kilometer race to raise money for a good cause. Just make sure that you're taking good care of yourself before you decide to devote more time to others.

Break Bad Habits

Some sneak up on you like a summer thunderstorm. Others take a lifetime to develop. But bad habits—from hair twirling to nail biting, from caffeine "addiction" to reaching automatically for an alcoholic drink at the end of the day—are not friends worth keeping.

What makes these seemingly innocent acts so bad for you? Some can slowly undermine your health. Others detract from your image as a mature person. Still others can mar your appearance. And let's not forget one other fact: Your bad habits likely get on other people's nerves.

Once you've developed a bad habit, it can be tough to shake—unless you know the practical secrets that can help you replace bad habits with healthy ones.

A Change for the Better

Regardless of why you picked up a particular habit, experts suggest a three-step approach for uprooting it once and for all.

- First, consciously realize you're doing it. Yes, that's *you* with your fingernail in your mouth. That's *you* drumming your fingers on the table at the weekly staff meeting.
- Second, determine what caused the bad habit to form in the first place. "If you don't, the chances are slim that you'll stop it, no matter how clever the remedy you try," says Andrea Van Steenhouse, Ph.D., a psychologist in Denver and author of *A Woman's Guide to a Simpler Life*.
- Third, take care of that underlying need by developing a new, healthy habit.

A word of advice: Be patient with yourself. It may take a few days or even a few weeks to free yourself completely from a bad habit, says Hyla Cass, M.D., assistant clinical professor of psychiatry at the University of California, Los Angeles, School of Medicine. But the results are worth it.

Here are some common nervous habits and expert-endorsed strategies for stopping them.

Alcohol Addiction

There's a world of difference between enjoying a drink and needing one.

Drinking too much—which experts say is more than 5 ounces of wine, 12 ounces of beer, or 1½ ounces of liquor in a day for women, about twice that for men—not only can lead to alcohol dependency but also puts you at higher risk for cancers of the stomach, esophagus, and breast. It may contribute to bone loss, raising the risk of osteoporosis. And if you're a woman who drinks two or three alcoholic beverages a day, you also raise your chances of developing high blood pressure by 40 percent, according to a 4-year study done at Harvard Medical School. Further, alcohol can reduce your body's ability to absorb fats and proteins as well as important vitamins and minerals such as folate and thiamin. This, in turn, can have serious effects on the brain, including memory loss, says Dr. Cass. In the short run, alcoholic beverages, particularly beer and red wine, are notorious for triggering headaches because they dilate blood vessels in your head.

To keep a bad habit from forming into a big problem, here's what to do.

Get some kudzu. Kudzu, a vine-sprawling legume, has been used in China for more than 1,300 years to discourage drinking and treat alcoholism. Studies show that two compounds in this herb, daidzein and daidzin, may be responsible for curtailing the desire to drink alcohol. For best results, take up to 100 grams of kudzu in capsule form a day (available in health food stores). Consult your qualified medical herbalist or physician for the right daily dose to meet your needs.

Try meditation. If you're looking to wind down, take a pass on the glass of wine and learn meditation. This ancient art of deep, slow breathing helps to calm your body naturally without the need for chemicals.

Caffeine Addiction

Can you remember the first cup of coffee you ever drank? Chances are you didn't instantly fall in love with it. But as the weeks and years passed, you acquired a taste for it. Now you may find that your relationship with coffee has become an obsession. In fact, you can't seem to function without that first, wake-me-up cup. Or the second. Or the third.

What's going on? Caffeine stimulates the central nervous system, which triggers the release of adrenaline and raises blood sugar levels. As a result, you feel more alert and focused. In the short run, caffeine lessens feelings of fatigue. But in the long run, too much coffee (or any other highly caffeinated beverage, such as diet cola) can lead to a condition called caffeinism (also known as coffee nerves).

The side effects of excess caffeine? You may feel lightheaded, fidgety, headachy, or a little nauseated. You may experience diarrhea, frequent urination, or insomnia. And that's not all. Too much caffeine may raise cholesterol levels and aggravate high blood pressure problems, premenstrual syndrome, and breast pain. It may put your bones at risk too.

"Besides possibly raising your cholesterol, caffeine also interferes with your body's absorption of calcium," cautions Judy Marshel, R.D., Ph.D., director of Health Resources in Great Neck, New York. "As women enter their forties and fifties, they need to be taking steps to make sure they are getting adequate levels of calcium to reduce their risk for osteoporosis—not preventing calcium from reaching their bones."

Take it slow. You can bid adieu to caffeine successfully if you wean yourself off it gradually. Give yourself a week to 10 days.

Stay clear of hidden caffeine. It may surprise you, but coffee isn't the only caffeine culprit. Chocolate, some iced teas, and sodas (including colas and some noncola soft drinks) also harbor high levels of caffeine.

Reduce your consumption ½ cup at a time. If you normally drink 4 or more sodas or cups of coffee a day, try cutting back by ½ cup every few days. Keep trimming back by ½ cup every few days to allow your body to adjust to the decrease in caffeine.

Flip-flop with decaffeinated coffee. After drinking a cup of regular coffee, make your second cup decaf. Keep alternating between the two. Gradually increase the number of decaffeinated cups and reduce the number of caffeinated cups until you are completely "decaffeinated."

Maintain your "coffee break" time. If you enjoy mid-morning and mid-afternoon breaks with your colleagues at work, continue this ritual, but simply switch your drink of choice. Fill your coffee cup with caffeine-free drinks such as bottled water, fat-free milk, or cranberry juice.

Limit to one. If you can't completely sever your caffeine ties, drink caffeinated beverages only when you really need to, such as in the morning for a wake-up energizer.

Finger Drumming and Toe Tapping

Maybe you possess a secret dream to be a band conductor. That may explain your need to drum your fingers on a tabletop, jiggle your knee while you sit in meetings, or tap your toes while you stand and wait for a bus. But more likely, boredom and stress account for these fidgety body motions.

Whether you're bored or not, finger drumming and toe tapping can deliver the wrong signals to others. Even if you don't say a word, your rhythmic tapping could be interpreted as a sign that you don't think what others are saying matters or is important. You won't win many allies that way.

Here's how to stop digits that fidget.

Join hands. The next time you feel the urge to tap out a rhythmic beat with your fingers, flash an image of a stop sign in your mind. Rest your hands in your lap, gently holding them together. You'll be more tuned in to what others are saying and less apt to annoy them with your finger strumming.

Watch yourself. Position yourself so that you can watch your reflection in a mirror or windowpane during a meeting.

Practice progressive muscle relaxation. Put your nervous energy or boredom into a healthy, no-sweat body workout. Start by tensing your forehead firmly for 10 seconds. Then release. Inhale and exhale slowly. Move down to your jaw, tensing and relaxing those muscles, and then to your shoulders. Systematically work your way slowly down to your feet. Remember to slowly inhale and exhale after relaxing each body part. You'll feel more relaxed.

Gum Chewing

Maybe as a child you could blow the biggest bubbles on your block. Or you sought to make the loudest smacks with each spit-filled chew. Years later, you chew and smack gum with regularity. Why? Maybe because you've grown accustomed to having something to chomp between meals. Or perhaps you fight nervousness and stress with gum-chewing workouts.

What you may not realize is that gum chewing can irritate coworkers and family members. Plus, you don't win many points for professionalism when you look like a grazing cow. Healthwise, if you are chewing lots of gum that's not sugar-free, you may be opening yourself up to dental problems such as cavities. So how can you break this rhythmic jaw-moving habit?

Suck on mints. If you like something in your mouth, switch to sugar-free mints. The taste will satisfy your oral needs, but sucking on these little candies won't result in decayed teeth as marathon gum chewing can.

Book a time. Schedule a 2-hour time slot each day to chew your favorite brand of gum. Ideally, pick a time when you're apt to be by yourself so your chewing won't annoy others, especially if you tend to make smacking noises.

Hair Twirling

Without realizing it, you automatically roll strands of your hair between your index finger and thumb. Close friends finally confide to you that your habit drives them crazy. Twirling your hair can distract you from stress, but it makes a grown person look 10 years old. What's worse, you could lose hair in spots, thanks to the pulling action.

Find a mirror. Sometimes, simple bad habits like hair twirling can be curbed by watching yourself do them. If you realize you're starting to twirl, find a mirror and watch yourself in action.

Reach for a smooth stone. For some people, hair twirling acts as a way to calm day-to-day anxiety. Try substituting a less noticeable soothing act, such as rubbing a smooth stone with your fingers. Keep one in your pocket or on your desk. Most folks won't notice your actions.

Nail Biting

Nibble, nibble, nibble, all day long. Every day you vow you'll stop biting your nails. But every day there's a snag or an uneven edge that begs for your toothy manicure.

Experts say nail biting is usually developed out of boredom or is a way to fend off stress. It's a definite habit to break for two reasons. Nail biting itself is unappealing, and it can also cause finger and nail infections because your mouth harbors germs that can be transferred to small tears in the skin around your nails.

Douse them in olive oil. Pamper split and cracked nails that beg to be bitten by dipping them daily in olive oil. Let your fingernails soak in a bowl with ½ cup of warmed olive oil for 15 to 30 minutes. Olive oil moisturizes and strengthens your nails naturally. The less brittle your nails, the less apt you are to bite them.

Keep clippers and files within reach. If you've snagged a nail while dressing, shut off the urge to conduct makeshift repairs with your teeth. Stock your bathroom, nightstand, purse, and car with fingernail clippers and emery boards. Keeping these finger tools within reach will help you smooth out the rough edges in a healthier and more attractive way.

Kill the bite urge with hot-pepper sauce. Or lemon juice. Or bitters. Anything that sends your tastebuds howling in protest can nip nibbling in the bud. These unappetizing finger dips should be applied daily until your nail-biting days are over—usually within 7 to 10 days. As a precaution, remind yourself not to rub your eyes or the skin near your eyes.

Reward yourself with a manicure and polish. Let a professional restore your bitten nails. Select a favorite fingernail polish hue for the finishing touch. "Nail salons are all over the place," says Dr. Van Steenhouse. "That first manicure may help restore pride in your nails. It's a healthy start to stopping nail biting."

Teeth Clenching

That clamped-jaw pose may convey toughness on the screen for Clint Eastwood, but teeth clenching can wreak Oscar-winning devastation on the enamel of your teeth.

"Pent-up stress is a major cause of teeth grinding and teeth clenching," says Elaine Kuracina, D.M.D., a doctor of dental medicine in Endicott, New York. Here's how to unclench and relax.

Maintain an air space. Unless you are chewing or swallowing, your upper and lower teeth should not touch. Make mental notes or post little reminders on your refrigerator, bathroom mirror, or near your desk at work reminding you to keep your lips together and teeth apart during the day.

Act like an NFL player. Wide receivers often wear mouth guards to protect their teeth from bone-rattling tackles. The same principle can assist you when you sleep. Try wearing soft plastic mouth guards while you sleep to keep your teeth from connecting. They are inexpensive and available at sporting goods stores.

Burn off some stress. Regular aerobic exercise—as little as 20 minutes three times a week—can help you relieve built-up stress and thereby reduce your tendency to clench your teeth.

Safe Use Guidelines for Herbs and Supplements

While taking vitamins, minerals, and herbs is generally safe, experts caution that you should use them responsibly. Foremost, if you are under a doctor's care for any health condition or are taking any medication, don't take any supplement or herb without your doctor's knowledge. Also, if you are pregnant, do not self-treat with any natural remedy without the consent of your obstetrician or midwife. The same goes for nursing mothers, women trying to conceive, and children.

Below are guidelines for remedies in this book that may cause adverse reactions. Such occurrences are rare, but discontinue use if you have an unusual reaction. Also, do not exceed recommended dosages.

By familiarizing yourself with this list, you can enjoy the world of natural healing with confidence.

Aloe: Do not use gel externally on any surgical incision because it may delay wound healing.

Arnica: Do not use on broken skin.

Black cohosh: Do not use for more than 6 months.

Black haw: If you have a history of kidney stones, do

not take without medical supervision because it contains oxalates, which can cause kidney stones.

Buchu: Do not use if you have kidney inflammation.

Cayenne: May irritate the gastrointestinal tract if taken on an empty stomach.

Chamomile: May trigger an allergic reaction in people allergic to closely related plants such as ragweed, asters, and chrysanthemums.

Chasteberry: May counteract the effectiveness of birth control pills.

Comfrey: For external use only. Do not use on deep or infected wounds because it can promote surface healing too quickly and not allow healing of underlying tissue.

Dong quai: Do not use while menstruating, spotting, or bleeding heavily since it can increase blood loss.

Echinacea: Do not use if allergic to closely related plants such as ragweed, asters, and chrysanthemums. Do not use if you have tuberculosis or an autoimmune condition, such as lupus or multiple sclerosis, because echinacea stimulates the immune system.

Eucalyptus: Do not use if you have inflammatory disease of the bile ducts or gastrointestinal tract or severe liver disease.

Fennel: Do not use medicinally for more than 6 weeks without supervision by a qualified herbalist.

Garlic: Do not use supplements if you are taking blood thinners because garlic thins the blood and may increase bleeding. Do not use if surgery is anticipated. Do not use if you are taking hypoglycemic drugs.

Ginger: Dried root or powder used in therapeutic amounts may increase bile secretions in people with gallstones. Fresh ginger is safe when used as a spice.

Ginkgo: Do not use if you are taking antidepressant MAO inhibitor drugs, aspirin or other nonsteroidal anti-inflammatory medications, or blood-thinning medications. In doses higher than 240 milligrams of concentrated extract, it can cause rash, diarrhea, and vomiting.

Ginseng: Do not use if you have high blood pressure.

Goldenseal: Do not use if you have high blood pressure.

Hawthorn: If you have a cardiovascular condition, do not take regularly for more than a few weeks without medical supervision. You may require lower doses of other medications, such as high blood pressure drugs. If you have low blood pressure caused by heart valve problems, do not use without medical supervision.

Horse chestnut: Can interfere with the action of other drugs, especially blood thinners. Can irritate the gastrointestinal tract.

Kava kava: Do not take with alcohol or barbiturates. Use caution when driving or operating equipment since this herb is a muscle relaxant.

Licorice: Do not use if you have diabetes, high blood pressure, liver or kidney disorders, or low potassium levels. Do not use daily for more than 4 to 6 weeks because overuse can lead to water retention, high blood pressure caused by potassium loss, and heart and kidney impairment.

Marshmallow: May slow the absorption of medications taken at the same time.

Parsley: If you have kidney disease, do not use therapeutically because parsley increases urine flow. Safe as a garnish or ingredient in food.

Peppermint: Ingestion of peppermint essential oil may lead to stomach upset in sensitive individuals. If you have gallbladder or liver disease, do not use without medical supervision.

Sage: In therapeutic amounts, it can increase the sedative side effects of drugs. Do not use if you have hypoglycemia or are undergoing anticonvulsant therapy. Safe when used as a spice.

St. John's wort: Can cause sensitivity to the sun. Do not use with antidepressants without medical approval.

Shepherd's purse: If you have a history of kidney stones, do not take without medical supervision because shepherd's purse contains oxalates, which can cause kidney stones.

Turmeric: Do not use therapeutically if you have high stomach acid, ulcers, gallstones, or bile duct obstruction. Safe for use as a spice.

Valerian: Do not use with sleep-enhancing or mood-regulating medications because it may intensify their effects. May cause heart palpitations and nervousness in sensitive individuals. If such stimulant action occurs, discontinue use.

Vitamin B_6: Doses above 100 milligrams must be taken under medical supervision because excess B_6 may lead to sensory neuropathy, with pain, numbness, and weakness in the limbs.

Vitamin C: Doses above 1,000 milligrams may cause diarrhea in some people.

Vitamin E: Although vitamin E is generally sold in doses of 400 IU, one small study showed a possible risk of stroke in dosages higher than 200 IU. Consult with your doctor if you are at high risk for stroke.

Zinc: Doses above 20 milligrams must be taken under medical supervision to ensure that copper intake stays in balance for proper immune function.

Index

Underscored page references indicate boxed text.

C

D

I

J

K

L

M